CROSSING BORDERS

CROSSING BORDERS

living and learning together
in a colourful world

by

Jenny Wickford

Fatumo Osman

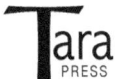

Crossing Borders
First Edition, 2018
Published by Tara Press
Dublin, Ireland

www.TaraPress.net

© Jenny Wickford and Fatumo Osman, 2018

ISBN: 978-1-9999262-2-9

This book is sold subject to the condition that it shall not, by way of trade or otherwise, be lent, resold, hired out, digitally reproduced or otherwise circulated without the publisher's prior consent in any form of binding, cover or digital format other than that in which it is published and without a similar condition being imposed on the subsequent purchaser.

Cover photo used with kind permission of Alisdair Miller www.AlisdairMiller.com

Book design: www.Cyberscribe.ie

FLOWERS ARE RED:
Words and Music by HARRY CHAPIN
© 1979 FIVE J'S SONGS.
All Rights Administered by WB MUSIC CORP. All Rights Reserved Used By Permission of ALFRED MUSIC.

A version of the "Reflective Framework" appeared in the European Journal of Physiotherapy 16:1, 41-48 and is reproduced with permission of Taylor & Francis, www.tandfonline.com

All proceeds from sales of this book will go directly to Noora Wellbeing, see: www.noorawellbeing.com

DEDICATION

for Myrra, Ilmi,
Nooria, Iro, Abraham,
Abdulahi, Juweria, and Ahmed:
you make our worlds colourful
may you grow up
daring to cross borders
seeing and valuing the colours
in this world

ABOUT THE AUTHORS

This book is written by us, Jenny Wickford and Fatumo Osman. We come from very different backgrounds but we also share experiences and thoughts about the world and what it means to live in it. We both grew up outside of Sweden, and we both moved to Sweden when we were 19. Jenny grew up in Pakistan, then moved to Sweden as this was the home country of her parents. Fatumo came to Sweden after fleeing from the civil war in Somalia.

Through sharing our stories, our experiences and thoughts, we formed an instant bond when we met. We realised that, as people, there were more similarities than differences between us. Even though our paths have taken different routes since we first met, we keep our common ground, and now, when we meet, we pick up the conversation where we left off. Part of this conversation we want to share with you in the pages that follow.

TABLE OF CONTENTS

preface 9

1 introduction 17

2 context 23

3 person 39

4 driving forces 49

5 participation 73

6 communication 85

7 reflection 101

8 collaboration 113

9 conclusion 119

epilogue 123

gratitude 125

chapter notes 129

bibliography and recommended reading 135

Preface

The world is more complex and colourful today than ever before. Human similarities are entangled with incalculable cultural, ethnic, religious and social diversities – and boundless individual variation. All this makes human encounters intriguing, educative and challenging when people migrate, for the reason of persecution, employment or love. For some, settling in a new place means tearing up their roots and putting their seeds somewhere else, to others getting new bearings in life, whereas to many it carries a sense of loss. For all of them, it is a border-crossing journey; familiarity and certainty is abandoned in the face of the unknown and unpredictable. This is when the ambiguous, vague and yet palpable thing we know as culture, is focal to our gaze. Language, norms, values, habits and ultimately the entire way we understand the world becomes visible. With the prospect of remaining who you think you are and yet becoming someone slightly different, migration is when our identity is at stake.

This is the essence of Fatumo and Jenny's book. With an analogy resembling the Spencerian one of society as an organism, and scientific concepts as their springboard, they shed light upon intercultural border-crossing and collaboration and how it enriches how we live and learn together. Vivid personal accounts and insightful reflections guide the reader on a journey where the meanings of person, context, communication, culture and the anatomy of intercultural interactions are addressed. For the reader, the book may be the beginning of a new journey of self-exploration and appreciation of human multiplicity. This is why I warmly recommend it.

Jonas Stier
Professor of Intercultural Studies
Dalarna University, Sweden

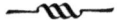

Prologue

A COLOURFUL WORLD

Flowers are red By Harry Chapin

The little boy went first day of school
He got some crayons and he started to draw
He put colors all over the paper
For colors was what he saw

And the teacher said, "What you doin' young man?"
"I'm paintin' flowers" he said
She said, "It's not the time for art young man
And anyway flowers are green and red"

"There's a time for everything young man
And a way it should be done
You've got to show concern for everyone else
For you're not the only one"

And she said, "Flowers are red young man
And green leaves are green
There's no need to see flowers any other way
Than the way they always have been seen"

But the little boy said
"There are so many colors in the rainbow
So many colors in the morning sun
So many colors in the flower and I see every one"

The teacher said, "You're sassy
There's ways that things should be
And you'll paint flowers the way they are
So repeat after me"

And she said, "Flowers are red, young man
And green leaves are green
There's no need to see flowers any other way
Than the way they always have been seen"

But the little boy said
"There are so many colors in the rainbow
So many colors in the morning sun
So many colors in the flower and I see every one"

The teacher put him in a corner
She said, "It's for your own good
And you won't come out 'til you get it right
And are responding like you should"

Well finally he got lonely
Frightened thoughts filled his head
And he went up to the teacher
And this is what he said

And he said
"Flowers are red, and green leaves are green
There's no need to see flowers any other way
Than the way they always have been seen"

Time went by like it always does
And they moved to another town
And the little boy went to another school
And this is what he found

The teacher there was smiling
She said, "Painting should be fun
And there are so many colors in a flower
So let's use every one"

But that little boy painted flowers
In neat rows of green and red
And when the teacher asked him why
This is what he said

And he said
"Flowers are red, and green leaves are green
There's no need to see flowers any other way
Than the way they always have been seen"

We both heard this song in different contexts, but it spoke to us of the same thing. What are we teaching our children about the world? Are we indoctrinating them with our own ideas, "the way they always have been", and with our own fear of that which is new or different? Are we limiting their natural curiosity and appreciation of the colourful diversity in this world? What kind of world will we create for our children, if we allow this to keep on going?

These are questions that we want to address in this book. We have no answers, and we don't think there is one answer. We only have our own personal lived experiences, our critical reflections based on these experiences, as well as on research and discussions, others' research, and others' experiences retold to us. The ideas developed from all this are conveyed herein, with the hope that others may be inspired to pause and think about their own colourful world, and their place in it. May we never stop appreciating and respecting the colours in the world!

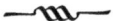

PART ONE:

The elements of borders

1 Introduction

CROSSING BORDERS?

> I have more respect for people who change their views after acquiring new information than for those who cling to views they held thirty years ago. The world changes.
>
> Michael Crichton (1)

Jenny:

People ask me where I am from, and my answer to this question never comes naturally. I was born in Sweden. I am Swedish for all official purposes. My parents are Swedish, both from the woods of Småland. I have inherited the local dialect from Småland, although I have lived there a very small percentage of my life. But I am not 'only' Swedish. I moved to Pakistan with my parents when I was five months old. I grew up in an international school in the foothills of the Himalayas in northern Pakistan, with people from all over the world. I then moved back to Sweden when I was 19, leaving my family and friends behind in Pakistan.

When I left Pakistan, my life as I knew it ended, leaving a hollow space in my heart. I gradually learned to live in my new country with its new culture. Yet part of that hollow space has remained, and it is best filled when I travel. Growing up in an international setting and moving often has made me into a nomad that feels most at home with people from different countries and backgrounds. I have thus continued to travel and cross borders, both within Sweden and internationally. Many personal and professional borders have also been challenged and crossed, since leaving Pakistan.

Living and working in different countries, getting to know people and their contexts in these countries, as well as working in different fields, have all been tremendous learning experiences. Ranging from factory work to teaching at university, from humanitarian development work in Afghanistan to clinical practice in the UAE, these experiences have been hugely fulfilling but never entirely easy. The travels, the very different contexts, cultures and people, have all contributed to broaden my understanding of this world we live in. They have shaped me as a person, and they have shaped my view of what it means to live together with other people in it.

Fatumo:

When people ask me where I come from my answer comes naturally. I am Somali born, from Mogadishu, and spent my first 19 years there. However, I am not 'only' Somali. I have lived in Sweden longer than I lived in Somalia. Therefore, both the Swedish and the Somali cultures have shaped me into who I am today. But the journeys I made have formed me as well; I fled from the capital, Mogadishu, at the beginning of the 1990s due to the civil war. I still remember the journey like it was yesterday; I was crossing Dolo, which is the border between Somalia, Ethiopia and Kenya. At that time, I was confronted with two choices – I could either go right to Ethiopia or left to Kenya. I chose left, to Kenya. I stayed in Kenya for almost a year before I left the Kenyan capital to find my way to Europe. During the time in Kenya I met different ethnic groups, learned the language and interacted with people who had different contexts and experiences than I had.

Sweden was not the destination that I had planned. I intended to reunite with my mother in France, but life chose a different direction for me. Today I am grateful for how it all played out. It was in Sweden that I started to reflect on my own culture and its meaning. I have crossed many borders in the past years that I have been living in Sweden, both within myself and within the country. I have gotten to know myself 'in-depth'. I have also crossed various professional borders, having worked as an interpreter, a volunteer in a primary school, a nurse in hospital and in the community, and now as a lecturer and researcher.

In 2011 I had the opportunity to go back to my country of birth. But this time it was to work on a development and education project. Combining the work I love, teaching and doing research, as well as being a part of my two countries, is what has shaped me into who I am today.

So, we have both crossed many borders in the time we have had thus far. Geographical borders, of course, but also professional borders and personal borders. Crossing borders is seldom easy, but it can be immensely rewarding and enriching. Crossing borders means meeting people from other cultures, with different traditions, practices and ideas. It means exposing yourself to the unknown, to uncertainty, to challenges. It also entails responsibility. There are various factors involved when working or studying in cultures and contexts other than your own. Or when living with people who have joined your context and culture.

We have both experienced moving to Sweden from other countries as young adults, but in very different ways. For Jenny, the practical side of moving to Sweden was easy; she had a Swedish passport and flew in on a plane. The emotional side was much more difficult. Being white and speaking a local Swedish dialect, she was treated as any other white Swede – yet on the inside feeling lost and lonely and very much alien to the context she found herself in. Being 'Swedish' was not something that came naturally, she did not want to be a Swede.

Fatumo had a very different route to Sweden, as described, fleeing to Sweden as a young, black, Muslim immigrant with a headscarf. She engaged with her new country, she learned the language fluently. She felt Swedish on the inside, but was treated as a foreigner. People still get surprised when she speaks fluently in Swedish.

Through these experiences, we have both developed a keen interest in what it means to live and work with people from different countries and cultures. Engaging with people from different cultures, in different contexts, we have become increasingly critical of the way in which the world is ordered and the manner in which we act towards each other. We live in a globalised world that is constantly changing and we want to inspire an interest and will to constantly develop ourselves and our ways of living, working and learning together in it.

Hence this book. We hope that it can be a support for those wanting to learn more about what it means to live in this world beyond the safe personal context.

About the book

This book is based on our personal experiences and perspectives and we use often personal experiences as examples. Our experientially influenced perspectives have been honed by much reading, studying, researching, reflecting, discussing and living in very different contexts. A number of authors that have been influential in shaping our ideas in this regard are listed at the end. We give these authors credit and thanks. Some parts of this book are also from Jenny's thesis (2).

There are also many people who have influenced us, and our views and beliefs. This book would not have happened without them. Everyone cannot be mentioned, but there are a few people who we would like to acknowledge, both for their impact on us personally, but also for their support and input into this book. These are also mentioned at the end of the book, in the chapter 'Gratitude'.

The book covers various components that play a part in how we live and learn together, in intercultural collaboration. There are two parts: the first part considers general components of collaboration, and the second part looks more specifically at how these translate into practical intercultural collaboration.

In addition to our stories, we use functions of the body to illustrate our points. We both work with people and with the human body. Jenny is a physiotherapist with the view that the complex individual cannot be understood out of its broader sociocultural context. Fatumo is a nurse with an interest in the holistic view of health. Thus we will use analogies from the body to exemplify aspects of collaboration.

This book is meant to be interactive. We do not have the answers to this very complex topic that we have broached – with no small measure of trepidation. We have lots of thoughts and ideas. But for this to mean something you need to think about it for yourself with regard to your own life. Thus, interspersed within the text are little reflections where you will be asked to reflect on what we've written in relation to your own life, beliefs and ways of doing things. These can also be used as a base for group discussions. As Kahlil Gibran said: "Knowledge of the self is the mother of all knowledge. So it is incumbent on me to know myself, to know it completely, to know its minutiae, its characteristics, its subtleties, and its very atoms" (3).

Read, interact, criticise, reflect, learn - and enjoy! At the end of the day, "all we have to decide is what to do with the time that is given us" (4), (wise words from Gandalf the Grey), so why not make it count for something greater than ourselves and our own little space in time?

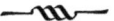

2 Context

DYNAMIC SYSTEMS OF PRACTICES

> Culture is to a human collectivity
> what personality is to an individual.
>
> Geert Hofstede (5)

Fatumo and Jenny have both done research and spent time in the academic world and in this context, have both learned the importance of definitions. Generally, people tend to use terms with an inherent, unconscious assumption that the person listening will have the same definition as us. In science, this assumption falls flat. Similarly, when talking to people from different backgrounds, traditions and cultures, the same issue arises (more on this in chapter 6). We may not be as clear as we think we are, based on how we use certain words.

Culture and context are two such terms that are used commonly in our everyday language. We will venture to say that we often assume we know what we mean, especially when it comes to a term such as culture. But when we ask people what they mean by 'culture', a clear definition rarely comes easily. We will therefore endeavour to look at culture and context from slightly different angles. But first we need base-line definitions.

> Reflection:
> How do you define context and culture?

Context and culture

Context, as it will be used here, is the immediate 'setting' we are in. It is the environment or social world in which we live, work and interact. It is not necessarily the national context, which can in fact be composed of several different contexts. If we say the context is the frame of the image of our lives at any given point in time and space, then culture adds colour to our thoughts and actions and practices within this frame. This is where it gets interesting.

Culture is a difficult term to nail down; discussed, disputed and varyingly defined. If, as Hofstede says, culture is what defines us as a collective body, then what is this culture? Importantly, when working with a term such as culture, one needs to arrive at a personal understanding. Our view is that cultures are dynamic and interdependent. They are learned – we are not born with a culture; we are born into a culture. Cultures can be re-learned and they impact individuals by comprising a framework within which individuals interact and learn social codes. At the same time, we shape cultures as we engage together in them. Culture is also unconscious and automatic. It reflects a perceived norm based on underlying values and assumptions about the world by a particular group. Values and beliefs are often taken for granted and it is when we are confronted with differences that our traditions and rituals can become more easily recognizable.

Cultures are thus defined as complex, diverse and dynamic systems of social meanings; as social frames of reference that are both constructed and affected by groups of people and affect the practices of these people. Culture is the medium through which people act and interact within the social world or context of which it is a part.

An important point to be made here is that culture cannot be used only in relation to people from other countries. Although cultural differences are often more blatant when individuals come from different countries this should not be assumed as the norm. There are often more similarities than differences. There are also many different subcultures within our own context. There may in fact be more differences between subcultures within a nation than between different national cultures. And what is this national culture? Is there such a thing as a national culture?

> Reflection:
> What is your culture? What are the aspects of your culture that you feel set you apart from someone else in your environment and where you think they are different?

Using the classic metaphor of the coin, we have cultural meaning on one side, and cultural practice on the other. If culture is the medium through which we act and interact, and our social constructions involve practices, then one could say that cultures are a collection of practices or a system of practices.

System of practices

When working with the body and its functions as a physiotherapist and a nurse, we view the body as a complex system that comprises a whole array of different parts and sub-systems that together make it a functioning, practicing whole. Our use of the terms 'practice' and 'system' are based on the following definitions: *Practice* is "the customary, habitual, or expected procedure or way of doing of something"(6). A *system* is "a set of things working together as parts of a mechanism or an interconnecting network; a complex whole; a set of principles or procedures according to which something is done." (7)

Each part of the human body can vary greatly, but each cannot function by itself. Essentially, we stay alive – and healthy – because all the cells in our body carry out their specific role, and importantly, they do this together with other cells, which might have radically different roles. It is the *system* of all these cells working together that makes the body function.

This system is made up of an intricate and fascinating array of cells that form complex structures, all held together by a network of connective tissue. Examples of these structures are bones, muscles, nerves, blood. Various combinations of these then comprise organs, and groups of organs make up subsystems. For example, we have the heart and the vessels, which comprise the subsystem called the circulatory system. Each organ and subsystem has various functions which we can call a practice. The practice of the circulatory system is to carry substances around the body that our cells need to survive, and to remove waste products no longer needed.

To carry out these practices, the organs or subsystems do not function by themselves. The practice of the circulatory subsystem needs to work together with other subsystems in the body. For example, simply put, the heart needs the collaboration of the myofascial (muscle and fascial) subsystem in getting the blood through the body; it needs the lungs to provide oxygen and remove carbon dioxide; it needs the gut to provide nutritional components. All these subsystems interact in the most amazingly complex way and, somehow, we take our body through life without disturbing these systems and their practices too much.

In a similar way, just as the body is a system made up of subsystems and components, each involved in specific 'practices', a social system is made up of an array of different cultural and traditional subsystems and practices. These social systems cannot exist without us individuals. We all have our own practices and, together with others, we form systems of practices. Through engaging in the world these practices change, whereby our system also changes, depending on our practices.

For example, taking another analogy from the body: how we use our bodies changes our bodies physically. If we keep our practice monotonous (such as sitting still for most of the day), our body-system will adapt to this. We will become more limited in what our bodies can handle, they will become more susceptible to damage. Our body-system will suffer the consequences and eventually our health will suffer too.

> Reflection:
> Make a note of practices that guide your way of living.
> What habits do you have and why?

What does this analogy mean on a social level? Our social systems of practices function best when all the individuals that are part of it have a role to play, and are given the agency and space to do so. Just as our bodies would be unable to exist if there was not the array of specialised cells doing their own thing yet together with others, a complex social system would not function well if people were not given the chance to participate in the system.

Just as we mentioned in the prologue, we need variety and colour in these systems. We need people who can do different things, and who have different perspectives. What will happen to our world, to our social systems, if we all start seeing flowers only as red and leaves only as green? Just as in the body, if we limit the practices of people in the system, then the system will adapt and become more limited. The social system will become more homogenous and lose its diversity and ability to meet a greater variety of demands. It will lose colour. The limitations will then affect the individuals in the system and what they engage in.

Finally, if one part or practice of the body does not function well, this will affect the functioning of the rest of the body. As the Prophet Muhammed, PBUH, said: *In the body there is a piece of flesh; if it is sound, the whole body is sound and if it is corrupt the whole body is corrupt.* In the same way a social system will be affected if one part of the system is not doing well. In mild cases, when something is not functioning as well as it could we can feel uncomfortable with the way things are but we are not in direct danger and the system doesn't fall apart (for example, patients whose social situation was the problem, not some dysfunction of their body). In extreme cases systems do fall apart, which leads to people having to leave their system and become refugees (as in Fatumo's experience).

Let's start with some examples of practices and systems and of how systems of practice impact and shape individuals. These are once again our stories based on our experiences and what we know, and this is just one perspective.

The practice of living in different systems

As mentioned in the beginning, we both grew up in countries other than Sweden. We will look more closely at how growing up in these different systems of practices, and then moving to other systems of practice, have impacted us.

Fatumo:

I was born and grew up in Mogadishu, the capital city of Somalia, located in the coastal Banadir region on the Indian Ocean. Growing up in this coastal city has had an impact on my life. I grew up in a country where the majority of the people shared one religion – Islam – one language with several dialects, and one ethnic group, with several clans. The religion of my parents and the society I lived in deeply shaped me and impacted my belief about morals and ethics. Tolerance and co-existence was something that I learned from my parents who were well educated and spent their lives in different countries. For my parents, education was not an option: it was a must, and they encouraged me to get an education and to be independent. My father passed away when I was 11 years old, so I had to take more responsibility and I grew up quicker than other girls my age. In secondary school I went to a school where all the subjects were taught in Arabic, all my teachers were Egyptians save the Somali literature teacher. I had a happy childhood despite all the responsibility I had as a first born child, where I had to help my mother take care of my siblings and be a strong role model for them. In school I was the bright and stubborn student who always followed her own way.

When the civil war started I began to question the values I had learned. I started to learn more about my religion and asked all the "why?" questions that any person who is curious would ask. We had the choice to either stay in Mogadishu or try to do something about the situation and flee. I fled from Mogadishu at the end of 1991 with my younger brother. We left the beautiful coastal city with a convoy of approximately 100 people heading to what we hoped was a safer place. But the road we took was not safe. On the convoy we were packed like goods: women, children and the elderly sat inside while the men and young boys sat on top of the convoy. It took five days to get to the border between Ethiopia, Kenya and Somalia. It was a trip I will never forget.

When we arrived in Nairobi we started another struggle; feeling safe and uncertain at the same time. Safe because we were finally out of the war, but uncertainty in the face of what our lives would be like in a country where we had no relatives. Our goal was to be reunited in France with our mother, but in the end, Sweden became the second home I never thought I would live in. Coming *to Sweden as an immigrant, learning the language, starting over with a new life and new dreams became a core part of my life. In the beginning, as I was learning about the new context I was in, the change in my being and mind started gradually without my even noticing it. By interacting with others I achieved an awareness of the structure of my own system, within the newness.*

As Hall (8) described, most cultural discovery starts with being lost. That is how I can describe my first years of living in Sweden. My habits from before started changing as I unconsciously started both to observe and imitate people around me, as well as become more aware of my own behaviour. In a system of practice I believe that you change your worldview and at the same time change the system you are a part of. My worldview today is the result of being part of several systems of practice, both past and present.

Jenny:

As mentioned earlier, I was born in Sweden, but when I was five months old my parents packed up their life there and moved to Pakistan. I then grew up being a part of two vastly different worlds in Pakistan and Sweden. Most of my growing-up years were spent in the stunning foothills of the Himalayas, with the green Scandinavian forests and lakes as an added heritage. I had the luxury of being able to move freely between these vastly different worlds. For example, during the first Gulf War the situation in Pakistan became more heated and we were evacuated – just in case. I remember the subsequent year we spent in Sweden, how it was uncertain when we could go back to Pakistan, and how intensely I wanted to 'go home'. Pakistan was my home, where I had my life, my friends. Sweden was the exotic place where we went on holiday.

After I graduated from High School, it was a difficult process moving back to Sweden. Sweden was strange to me. I could not relate to the social habits of people I met. I didn't like the language

(*English was my language of preference*). I missed my friends and family and the life I had with an intensity that left me feeling hollow. It took me several years to reconcile with my Swedish identity and heritage.

As an adult, I have continued to travel, and as mentioned, have lived in different places and different countries. Most of my life has thus been spent away from Sweden, with people from a diverse range of countries. The person I am today is a result of growing up in an international setting comprising many different practices, then continuing to take part in different systems of practices as an adult. The beliefs I grew up with have deeply impacted my principles and views about morals, ethics, and the responsibility we have for how we treat each other, ourselves, and the world we live in. Through personal experience, mistakes, challenges and reflections, I continue to become more aware of my own role, beliefs and values. Based on all this I've developed a set of practices that are a core part of my life. I take these practices with me into the different contexts I am in. These practices are not static, and these are adapted through interaction with others, and together we impact the systems of practice we are in.

For example, in the United Arab Emirates (UAE) I came into the job with slightly different clinical practices than those in place. I worked with a group of therapists from different countries. We shared a similar base but we had variations in our ways of being physiotherapists. As I learned more about the context I was in I both adjusted my own practice as I learned the new codes (often through making mistakes!), but also brought change to the practice I was in. This is true for anyone who participates in and engages in a practice. In the end I had a tremendous learning experience and came away with different nuances to my practices than when I arrived.

We have had different experiences on our journeys to becoming 'Swedish'. We have also found much common ground. We both grew up in contexts that are very diverse. We both crossed country borders, but we also crossed personal borders; we have developed our practices with influence from our parents, from the contexts that we have lived in and the people we have interacted with. Consciously and unconsciously we have changed our worldviews; even as we write this book our worldviews are dynamically changing, with every new experience.

Living in different systems, developing and becoming part of different practices, is done together with others. We were both affected by the experiences we had growing up, and through moving from one context to another, very different one. We found common ground through our experiences, even though the only major commonality in our experiences was moving to Sweden when we were 19. Despite the differences we found we had many similar thoughts about what we had been through.

Having said this, we do not imply that it will always be the case. Other people with the same experiences would have responded in different ways depending on their personality, genetics, and the people they spent time with. Sharing similar histories does not mean we will find it easier to 'connect' and understand each other. As an example, we look at the way Sweden has changed the past few years, and hear story after story of people who have grown up together but come out with radically different views on how we should treat the stream of immigrants that have been fleeing from their war-torn countries. Context and culture are only one component, there are other factors that impact who we are and how we interact, some of which we will look at in the next two chapters.

In relation to coming into a new context, we both came into vastly different systems of practices than we had known before, and we share the perception that we were expected to shed our previous ways and embrace the new. However, the expectations we perceived were – and are – very different. Our different skin colours, our ways of dressing, our manner of speaking all triggered different responses from people. For example, Jenny was often asked rhetorically, "Isn't it wonderful to be home"? Which she has always found strange, because for a long time, home was not Sweden. Fatumo's children are constantly asked where they come from even though they were born in Sweden.

Fatumo:

My children have given up constantly having to explain that they are from Sweden. The other day my daughter told me that she says, "I came to Sweden 18 years ago" She uses her date of birth as the time she came to Sweden and to the world.

Another example pertains to language and context. Even though Jenny spoke Swedish fluently with a local accent when she moved back to Sweden, she sometimes said things that were slightly eccentric or mispronounced, as she didn't have the same cultural background and experience with the language. Sometimes she did things that were slightly 'out of the box'. But in these cases her ways of speaking or acting were seen as quirky blunders. She was a 'Swede'. When Fatumo made a similar language or behavioural blunder that was not in line with the cultural framework she perceived that it was judged negatively as a cultural mistake. Granted, our understanding of how others perceived us was impacted by how we viewed ourselves in the new places and situations were in.

We all put people in boxes. We judge people by how they act, how they dress, how they speak. It is believed that people often react negatively when things are not according to their system of practice. They are on a so-called cultural autopilot and derive interpretations according to their belief of how people 'should' act in a particular culture or context.

One central concern here is the risk of dichotomizing people into 'us' and 'them' or 'others'. We think and act on the base assumption that we have more similarities with people like 'us' and more differences with the people that are not like us, the 'others'. From our experiences this is a false and misleading assumption. We are actually likely to have a poor and limited understanding of what 'we' are, unless we have spent time trying to understand this. 'We' are quick to judge anyone outside of our own group. Some or all of our (mis)understanding of so-called 'others' may be built on false, prejudicial and stereotypical information. People always have a reason for doing what they do and we should be very careful not to judge before talking to them and finding out their perspective, and before reflecting over why we react the way we do.

This doesn't mean we will always reach common ground, or that reaching common ground is necessarily the goal. It does not imply that cultural relativism is the way to go. But we have a responsibility for how we do things, how we act towards others, how we treat them. We'll discuss this more in the second part of the book.

We are creatures of adaptability. We have adapted through the centuries. Our systems and our practices are not static; they never have been. They will keep changing, as the world keeps changing. Let's not be so narrow-minded that we cannot learn from each other and be open to change.

> Reflection:
> How are you affected by different contexts you are in?
> Different countries? The city? The countryside?
> Forests? Noisy restaurants?
> What do these contexts do to you? How do you feel?

Dynamic systems

As we live and learn, we change. We, Jenny and Fatumo, are not the same persons we were at 20. As we engage in others' lives we have an impact on each other. As we engage in groups, our collective practices gradually mould and shift based on the people in the practice: some people stay for long, new people join the practice, some people leave. As we are confronted with issues and situations that challenge our ideals and morals, we can either stick our heads in the sand or we can learn from them. As we learn we impact the practice and the people around us – leading us to think about the dynamics of such systems.

A dynamic system changes over time. It changes when the components and practices of the system change. Sweden is not the same place it was 50 years ago. Neither is Somalia, Pakistan, Afghanistan nor the UAE. The systems are dynamic and interactive – they *change*.

Let's start with another illustration from the body. When Jenny meets a client an important part of the assessment is talking about past and current practices, habits, accidents, surgeries, movement behaviours, work etc. All this information is used to guide the subsequent physical assessment. Putting it all together, she can make a hypothesis about what is going on and what actions could be taken to improve the situation. There are factors that cannot be accounted for and this is true in any system. But by making a thorough assessment about what has happened before, what is going on now, and by establishing the level of function of the different body systems in relation to the practices of these systems, a plan can be made to get the body-system running as smoothly as possible in relation to the client's context.

The above treatment process usually takes time and commitment. It seems that often, instead of doing a holistic assessment of the situation that might entail working with life-style changes that can take a long time, we opt for quick fixes that don't deal with the root of the problem. Things settle for a while, but then the problem comes back. We brush over it, leading to a cycle of 'copy paste repeat'. How long can we keep doing this before things start breaking down and we need more drastic repair measures?

The same thing happens with our social and cultural systems of practices. How often do we opt for quick social or political solutions that do not take into consideration the complex dynamic system of practices? If we describe the current cultural context, the dynamic system of practices, and look at where we have come from, then we can hope to get a better understanding of where we are at present and where we are heading. We all have a past and a present. Do we blunder blindly into the future or do we consciously try to learn from the past by putting this together with the present and try to see where we are going? We would say that on the large scale of society and of the world, we do this poorly. We make the same mistakes that we did last year. But this can change. We have so much to learn from where we have been and where we are now to guide where we are going. To do this we need to learn to listen, to look, to reflect, and to have the guts to make the changes.

Despite how logical this appears on paper, it seems hard to do in practice. Again, we fall back on our experiences as examples. First, Afghanistan: more than 15 years after the fall of the Taliban the situation in Afghanistan is far from stable. Owing to many years of drought and destruction the country is run down on all levels and is rearing a generation that has known only war and displacement. Since the fall of the Taliban it has been the recipient of massive military intervention and support, humanitarian aid, emergency relief and development efforts, all from a broad array of international governments, donors, agencies and non-governmental organizations (NGOs). Although there has been progress in many sectors since 2001, despite all the above input Afghanistan remains one of the least developed countries in the world. Furthermore, despite massive international development, peacekeeping and military efforts, the security situation has steadily deteriorated. Afghanistan was not always like this. Jenny remembers stories growing up where people told of holidays spent in Kabul, as it was more modern than the cities in Pakistan.

The example of Somalia is very similar to the one from Afghanistan. More than 25 years after the fall of the Siad Barres regime the situation is far from stable in many places in Somalia. Owing to many years of civil war, conflicts, drought and destruction, Somalia has been and still is the recipient of massive military intervention and support, humanitarian aid, emergency relief and development efforts, all from a broad array of international governments, donors, agencies and non-governmental organizations (NGOs). The Somalia of today is not the Somalia Fatumo knew as a child: *I grew up in Mogadishu, called "the white pearl" in the late 70s and early 80s. Mogadishu was named one of the best and safest cities in Africa. Now it is one of the most devastated and dangerous cities in East Africa.*

We both wonder how such a mess could be made, even after all the years of experience from other countries and other wars? We, Jenny and Fatumo, came out of our years in Afghanistan and Somalia rich with personal experience but deeply disturbed by the way development work is practised. We don't understand how so many mistakes are made – despite all the years of knowledge to draw on – leaving these countries worse off than before. Where is it ever going to end?

Unfortunately, Afghanistan and Somalia are not the only cases. The current situation in the world, with 'terrorism', rising problems of racism (or the uncovering of previously-veiled racism), islamophobia, afrophobia and animosity toward immigrants, seem to imply that we haven't learned from previous mistakes.

Have we lost track of where we started? How do we describe our current system of practices and who defines this? How do we collectively understand these systems of practices so that we can see where we are going, make changes necessary to ensure that we are building a world we actually want our children to live and grow old in?

A system of practices can only exist because we create it. Any breakdown in the system happens because we are not taking care of the smooth running of the practices. We are not ensuring that the practices are functioning as a greater whole. Because we make the systems of practices, we need to look closer at who we are, and what drives us. This will be considered in the next two chapters of this section.

3 Person

PERSONAL PRACTICES AND STATES OF BEING

> Study me as much as you like, you will never know me,
> for I differ a hundred ways from what you see me to be
>
> Rumi

Jenny:

In my practice as a therapist I see it as absolutely essential that you, as my client, take an active role in any treatment measures taken. I want you to learn more about your body, to understand better why things may not be working the way they should, why you might need to make changes in your lifestyle. Quick fixes are doubtful considering the complex body that works as a whole. Short-term relief is not the goal. Long-lasting, healthy, functional systems are.

For this to work you probably need to make some changes in your life. This can only start with you. You need to want to understand your own movement behaviour, your habits and ways of dealing with stress, emotions etc. You need to have a basic understanding of how your body functions and responds to how you use it. You will need to understand your personal practice, and its impact on you as an emotional and physical system of practices. You will need to understand the importance and impact of context on how you as an individual function. If you cannot understand your body and why it is doing what it is doing, it is going to be hard to make any changes that will make it function the way it should, in harmony with its potential.

This is not so different from what it means to understand oneself in relation to understanding how we function together with others in our joint systems of practices. The individual person is the smallest entity in a community. The collection of individuals creates social norms, traditions and cultural practices. We all have our own personalities and identities, but we are social beings and we affect, and are affected by, those around us. If we are not functioning well, we will affect those around us. When this adds up, our practices and systems of practices start being affected.

We quoted Rumi above who said that you can never fully understand another person. But we can try – we should try. We are inherently social beings and creating meaning is the heart of the human experience. We always interpret others based on who we are, and others will respond to us based on how we act. So, the first step in understanding others is that we have to start with ourselves. We will look more closely at how to do this practically in Part II, but first we need to start with taking a look at who we are as individuals, and why.

Personal practices

Much has been written about the person as an individual, how we perceive the world, what makes us who we are. Many others have written better analytical accounts and theoretical descriptions about who we are and why we do what we do. For example, see meaning perspectives and transformative learning as described by Mezirow (9). We are going to discuss who we are and why in terms of the personal practices that we all have.

As we saw in the last chapter, a practice is by definition something that we do regularly, and with the aim of getting better at it. The practices we choose to engage in are based on the habits, preferences and skills that we have developed in interaction with others as we grow up. We are born with certain characteristics but the static nature of these is greatly questioned. Just as with the rest of our body, our DNA is affected by our experiences, by how we use our bodies. We develop our characteristics through our experiences and through our participation in the contexts we engage in (see more chapter 5).

Jenny had the privilege of growing up with an array of different people from different countries, both from living in Pakistani communities and living closely with people from different countries in an international school. She grew up with parents who believed in doing good in the world, in helping others, who were adventurous and took her and her siblings along on their adventures. Fatumo grew up with parents who pushed her to develop her potential, who believed in the importance of education. As a teenager, she took responsibility for her siblings when her father passsed away. And as a teenager she had to flee her home, and together with her brother, take full responsibility for her own life. She also had the opportunity to live with people from different countries during her stay in the refugee camp in Sweden. Very quickly she found a common ground with those people. The refugee camp was her first picture of Sweden: where different people could live together no matter where they came from. Has this picture changed?

Fatumo:

Even if the same picture still exists in my mind, I sometimes feel that various political influences and the rhetoric that some politicians and media use against certain groups in society, challenges coexistence and creates mistrust and tensions between people. However, it is our aim with this book to encourage people to start reflecting on, and critically questioning, these issues. We want to live in a colourful, diverse world. We want to seek knowledge within ourselves but also around us and around the world. My grandfather used to recite what the Prophet Mohammed PBUH said: "seek knowledge even in China". What Mohammed meant was, naturally, not China in particular, but rather that people should go far away to get knowledge from others. This saying followed me through childhood and into adulthood.

Our different experiences have naturally shaped who we are as adults and the choices we have made. But this doesn't stop just because we have grown up. We have developed a state of being that continually develops and changes throughout life and that impacts how we develop and change. As we described previously, we develop movement behaviours that will impact the shape and form of our body. If you spend most of your waking time sitting, then your various body tissues will adapt to this, leading to physical changes that in turn will impact how you are able to move. If you do not see this as an issue, if you do not want to change your movement behaviour, or understand how your body is interacting with the environment, then you will continue in the same movement behaviour. In the same way, if you have a habit of judging people in a certain way, or of reacting in a certain way, you will never change unless you are able to take a critical look at yourself and try to see why you react the way you do.

We know that most people perceive their own personal practices as normal. This is not a problem unless it is extrapolated to your own culture and system of practices being the 'norm' by which others should be judged. With this approach you will not be able to understand why situations happen the way they do or why people react to you the way they do. Not unless you take a good look at your manner of behaviour, your attitudes, your personal practices. We are complex beings, and we have so many sides that merit getting to know.

Layers

If anyone has seen a documentary about the internal body, or perhaps observed an operation, you will know the complexity that lies beneath the surface of the skin. We walk around with the most incredible, amazing complexity. A whole world exists inside us, yet on the outside all we see is the skin. Skin that comes in a myriad of different colours. But this colour is found only in the very outermost layer of the skin. Beneath this, we all have the same arrangement of structures, layers that can be differentiated with a scalpel but that are also intricately part of one another: the layers of the skin, the superficial fascia, the deep fascia, the muscles, the organs. These are intricately linked together by connective tissue, nerves, vessels.

We are all layers. Layers upon layers, upon layers. Our layers are all part of each other. One does not exist without the other. We put a lot into our layers. Experiences, good and bad, help shape who we are. We expose different layers to different people. Different layers will come into play in different situations with different people, depending on our emotional state, our relationship with others, our beliefs – both in general and in relation to what we are experiencing. Our outer layer, the one the world sees, is really not much to go on. As we get to know people we realise that the outer layer does not say much about the complex and beautiful being that exists beneath the surface.

Just as we affect our body-layers depending on how we use our bodies, we affect our personal being-state layers depending on how we deal with the experiences we have.

Being-states and world-views

We have borrowed the term 'state' from physics, where different states are what describe a system. We have particular states of being that impact how we engage in the world around us, how we interpret our experiences, how we engage in our practices.

These states of being, or being-states, are directly impacted by an array of different forces that are at work at any given moment (more on this in the next chapter). Our being-states are a direct result of our upbringing. The way our brain functions is dependent on the level of stimulation we received as children, the type of education we received, the amount and type of physical activity we engaged in. Our brains' functions are in direct interaction with our emotional and hormonal states. So our being-states are a result of these different parts of our body-systems. Our being-states comprise the perspective with which we engage in social activities, participate in the world, and learn. How we solve problems defines much of what we learn and how open we are to learning. This is again dictated by the state of being with which we approach these problems.

Being-states are not static. Just as our brains are not static but change based on how we use them, so our states of being change; they change depending on how we engage with people around us. We also change depending on how we deal with life and situations that we go through. As they say, situations can make us or break us.

Interlinked with our being-states is our world-view. By world-view we mean that each individual has their own perception and preferences about the world, how they navigate social situations, and how they interpret others' actions and their own experiences. Your perception, attitudes, preferences and expectations have developed through your being-state interacting with the world. It is the sum of the knowledge you have from participating – living and learning – in the world. It shapes our expectations of the world.

For example, before Fatumo came to Sweden and experienced the cold and the snow, one of her relatives who visited London in the 1980s told her that whenever it snowed in London, nobody went to work or school. She believed that, and thought it would be the same in Sweden. When she came to Sweden and experienced her first snow, she was surprised when she was told that everybody goes to work or school whether it snows or not. The expectations she had were developed by someone else in a different context. It was not until she engaged in her own context that she was able to find sense in it. With her experiences she now has developed different expectations.

Although the above is a simple example, it illustrates how quickly we can judge based on what we are told rather than what we experience for ourselves. In the same manner, we create perceptions of other people that we assume are not like us. Without knowing them, but based on what we have experienced and heard before, we make assumptions that they behave in a way that's either 'good' or 'bad' (as per our own definition). We thus create world-views – either rooted in experience or through what we hear and read from others.

Just as our being-states change, these world-views change along with our experiences, life situation, education, cultural and social structures etc. Importantly, they change through interacting with others. How this can change constructively is something that we will come back to later in the book.

Let's go back to the example of patients who come for treatment. Many of these come due to back pain. Commonly, this is a result of life-style and movement behaviour that slowly but surely wears the body down. Some people come and expect to be 'healed'. They want a quick fix with as little personal responsibility as possible. It doesn't matter if this is the fifth time their back seizes up. On the other end of the scale there are those who come in and realise that unless they use the current state of pain to gain a better understanding of themselves and and why they keep getting back pain, they will not get better in the long run. The latter are easy to work with. The challenge is the former, to understand their perspective and find a way to work with them that can lead to sustainable health changes.

Often, times of pain are a wake-up call, a time to take a look at what we are doing, or how we are living. This does not only relate to bodily pain. It could be a burn-out, losing a job, being forced to leave our home, losing someone we love, or falling out at work. The difficult times we go through, be they physically, emotionally or financially painful, can be the means to develop more tools and a greater appreciation for what life has to offer. *This is not easy.*

When she left her life in Pakistan behind and went to Sweden, Jenny wrote a series of poems as one way to deal with the loneliness and the loss. When Fatumo read the poems she felt they described her emotional experiences as well. Sharing these stories was thus both a way to heal and a way to share understanding. From the prologue: *"Life is not easy. It rarely takes us where we expected. But when it comes down to it, life is beautiful, and the grey times that we go through can bring out the depth and intensity of the colours that we had, all along."* (10) We believe this, but having both gone through various difficult times in life, we know it is hard. To learn through living doesn't come easily. Finding our colours, seeing new colours, takes work.

Also, we all have different genetic make-ups that give us different tools with which we engage differently in our experiences. Our bodies are different and react differently to the same types of forces being subjected to it. Some people are more prone to stress than others. Some are more prone to developing back pain. Just as people react to pain differently, and take responsibility for their dysfunctions differently, people react to life differently. We are who we are in interaction with the environment, but we also have certain bases that are ours genetically from our parents. We're not going to delve into the whole discussion about nature versus nurture, but just as the body has its specific characteristics, so do our personalities, our ways of being in the world. We, Jenny and Fatumo, are both fairly critical people by nature, who strive to understand and find solutions, and we thrived in educational and university environments that enabled us to develop this. Our classmates, who went through the same processes that we did, developed various skills – similar or different – depending on the skills they brought with them, and how they interacted with the systems we were in.

So, in following this reasoning, it can be said that we are somewhat limited by our own being-states. In other words, we will interpret our surroundings based on all that we already believe and hold true, as suggested by Rumi in the quote in the beginning of the chapter. But this is far from static, and we can consciously work on this. Although we can never truly know another person we can endeavour to try. We need to understand ourselves and why we interpret others and their actions the way we do. In this respect, it becomes of great value to interact with people who don't confirm what we already hold to be true, but who can challenge what we believe and thus facilitate a development and change in our being-states and our world-views. We will develop this further in the next chapter, regarding what it is that drives us and that drives change.

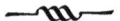

4 Driving forces

PUSHING, PULLING OR STATUS QUO?

> Fear is the mind-killer. Fear is the little death that brings total obliteration. I will face my fear. I will permit it to pass over me and through me. And when it has gone past me I will turn to see fear's path. Where the fear has gone there will be nothing. Only I will remain.
>
> Frank Herbert (11)

Without forces, the world would stop moving.

In our work as healthcare professionals, it never fails to amaze us how the body works based on, and in response to, the forces it is subjected to. The great majority of us give little thought to the complexity of forces at play in our bodies every breathing second. We rarely stop and consider how we use and abuse our bodies, and how the forces involved have an impact on a cellular level, so that we physically change as a result.

When it comes to the physical environment around us we have learned to use and harness forces to achieve a whole array of wondrous creations. We have identified atoms and electrons and magnetic fields. We have developed our understanding of how forces make the world go around and use this understanding to do amazing things, like fly and go into space. Jenny would never have thought, when she was ten and spoke on a crackling telephone line to her grandparents, that she would in a couple decades be able to talk to her family live on a computer, as if they were sitting across from her.

But what about the forces that drive us to act in different ways? What about the forces at play just under the surface in any interaction between people? How much do we consider these? These are the forces we will consider in this chapter.

Forces

Again, let's start with the definition. A force is, very simply, a push or a pull. Balanced forces on an object equal no movement of the object; unbalanced forces on an object will result in the object moving. Thus, objects in the everyday world (where friction operates) either stay put, are pushed or pulled. There is a whole array of different forces but for the present argument, only the general idea of a force is needed.

As a physiotherapist, forces help Jenny understand how the body works, how various forces can be used or misused to support or overload the body:

Jenny:

I consider forces when looking at movement, holding patterns and exercise positioning. I base my understanding of movement and its impact on the body on the idea that the forces we subject our bodies to, shape and mould them over time. By trying to balance and vary forces the aim is to avoid overload, underload or compensation. Forces can also be used more directly with manual applications to soft tissues: applied force (pressure), friction (rubbing), tension ('stretching'), to name a few. Although the manner by which – and if – this works is disputed, direct manual interaction has an impact on the individual. We only have theories for what happens, but whether impacting the body through manual techniques or through movement, we can feel something change. The forces we subject the body to leads to change.

Fatumo has pondered forces related to psychological, mental and spiritual areas:

Fatumo:

Leaving Somalia involved a strong push factor for me. This major force that caused me to leave my country was the combination of war, violence and lack of stability that was going on during that time. I had never wished to or dreamt of leaving my country. My dream was to go to medical school and become a doctor like my father. Those forces (war, violence and lack of stability) pushed me to make a dangerous journey, which is something I tend to forget now, so many years later. Another example of forces is how I constantly have to fight to show that I am a part of the Swedish society and community. I am never in 'status quo'. I am always pushing or pulling. But don't take this as something negative: as a reader, you might think, "what a struggle!" But I have never viewed these forces as a struggle. Rather, I see them as constructive forces that continuously help me to move on and become a better person.

In our interactions with each other there is an impact on us emotionally, psychologically, mentally, spiritually – and in turn, these can also cause physical changes in our bodies. Some people are more sensitive to this than others and will pick up on the nuances and undertones in the interaction. But few people can go through life and be immune to the impact of other people on their lives.

We talked about being-states in the previous chapter.

Our current being-state is dependent on all that we have experienced before. It is in constant interaction with our current system and practices. So just as the physical body will be impacted by the various forces subjected to it, so the emotional, mental, psychological body will change, based on the input coming in. (See 'The brain that changes itself' in the reference list at the end for a great book on this topic!). We will call these the forces of human interaction.

> Reflection:
> Think back on your life. Can you identify times and situations that have had an impact on you as a person? How and why did they have an impact on you?

Forces of human interaction

The challenge with forces of human interaction is that they are never constant. They will be different in different people, at different times in their lives, and in different contexts. As discussed in the previous chapter, we will interpret the world around us based on our personal understanding that has developed from our personal experiences. Despite all this, here is a tentative try at defining forces of human interaction.

Ultimately, there are two general reasons for doing what we do: either for our own gain or for the other's benefit. In between, there is a grey zone where we have mutual gain. Thus, we can place these two points on each end of a continuum, where any action that we take lies somewhere along these lines. Where on the continuum depends on which force is greater: the pulling force of personal gain or the pushing force of other's benefit.

Personal gain ─────────── Other's benefit

If we are completely honest with ourselves, how much of what we do is altruistically, solely for the benefit of the other, without any added benefit for ourselves, whether the belief of rewards in heaven, karma, or for simply feeling better about ourselves? We do not believe these are bad incentives/motives, but we do believe that it is useful to be honest with ourselves about why we do the things we do. Having said this, there are numerous stories of people who, when suddenly faced with the imminent danger to others' lives, reflexively and instantly engage in trying to save others. So, when there is no time for our being-state to consider the matter at hand in light of personal impact or gain, and we act on instinct, how many of us would risk our own lives for those of others? Are we more humane when we remove the filter of conscious thought?

Conversely, when we have time to think about things, how much of what we do is truly self-less? How much is a conscious weighing of pros and cons? Which is greater, the push or the pull? We will come back to this in the chapter about reflection, but for now, here is an example from Fatumo's experience:

Fatumo:

We often do things because we also have something to gain. For example, I have been involved with a project with Dalarna University collaborating with universities in Somalia, to provide a Master's Programme for Midwives in Somalia. Midwives who graduated from the programme were qualified to teach future midwives and in such a way reduce the extreme shortage of midwifery teachers and midwives that exists in the country. The projects are now completed and I can more easily look back and see what it was that drove my involvement and participation.

I was glad to be a part of the project for two reasons: it involved both personal gain and other's benefit. Personally, I would once again see my country, I would help my people, which has been a dream for a long time. Most of all I would get the opportunity to give support from my second home, Sweden. It would also be beneficial for Somalia to get midwife teachers and more midwives, and for Dalarna University to get the opportunity to develop an exchange both culturally and professionally. The driving forces for this work were thus beneficial on many levels, both for myself and others. This drove me and gave me the power to work late nights and do overtime. It enabled me to do more than was expected of me, to drive the partners in different institutions (both Somali institutions and Dalarna University) to develop strategies that were beneficial for all parties.

Power

An important 'force' to consider is the one of power. Working together with other people there will always be some form of power play. We need to look at how we create these plays of power and how they can impact our work.

By pure definition, power is not a force. It is however, related to forces. Power is the energy involved in forces moving objects. In physics terms, power = work per unit time, i.e. power is the result of how much energy is consumed in a certain given amount of time. As a noun, power is "the ability or capacity to do something or act in a particular way; the capacity or ability to direct or influence the behaviour of others or the course of events; physical strength and force exerted by something or someone" (12).

Power in our discussion here is the measure of how much I, as one individual, am able to move you, as another individual, to do what I want you to do, or vice versa. If we put this into our continuum above, power is related to where along the line we place ourselves based on the reasons behind our actions towards others. When the pushing and pulling forces are equal between personal gain and others benefit, then the power is mutually shared. The closer we get to personal gain, the greater our power; the closer we get to other's benefit, the less power we have. Yet it is not quite this simple because on the other hand, when helping others, do we gain some manner of control over them and thus more power?

This is clearly not simple, and we acknowledge that we are presenting a severe simplification of a subject that is inherently complex. But as our aim is not to delve into theoretical intricacies but to stimulate a discussion and reflection about what drives us, we suggest that this can suffice to bring to light what might be going on when we act in a certain way. Again, let us give some examples from our own experiences and lives in relation to working as a development worker in Afghanistan and to coming to Sweden as a refugee.

Power is an inescapable component of social interactions. People create cultures, and the way in which power is used in these social interactions can be characteristic of a specific culture. Geert Hofstede (13) has done some interesting work on culture. He has rated a number of countries based on different dimensions: power distance, uncertainty avoidance, individualism versus collectivism, masculinity versus femininity, and long-term versus short-term orientation. Somalia and Afghanistan are not included in his list, but Pakistan and the Arab Emirates are, as is Sweden. The Power Distance Index (PDI) varies between these countries. Power distance is "the difference between the extent to which [the boss] B can determine the behavior of [the subordinate] S and the extent to which S can determine the behavior of B" (13, p.83). For example, high PDI involves strong hierarchies with vertical power structures, whereas low PDI contexts have more horizontal power structures. Pakistan (PDI 55) and Arab countries (PDI 80) rate high on the scale. Sweden, on the other hand, has a low PDI of 31, as do various other European countries (13, p.87).

Even though Afghanistan is not described by Hofstede, these dimensions inspired thoughts about the work Jenny was involved in in Afghanistan:

Jenny:

I was a young unmarried female physiotherapist and research student who had left her family and travelled alone to the other side of the world to live and work in Afghanistan where age is honoured, collectivity is valued, marriage is the norm, and where women at large are not highly educated or proactive in the public or work arena. As an outsider/newcomer from a high income country and with a privileged education, I engaged in teaching and promoting professional development of physiotherapists from a different culture, religion and background, all within the Afghan development context.

What implications did this have for the work? As mentioned, cultures with a high PDI generally have strong hierarchies, and hierarchies were part of the Afghan context. Furthermore, the development context reinforced the hierarchical systems. Being part of this context, the potential of power that came along with Jenny's position naturally had consequences for her role and identity.

As a development worker Jenny was employed to teach and work toward improving and strengthening the physiotherapy services in the programme, and this placed her in a particular position in relation to her Afghan colleagues:

Jenny:

I had knowledge to share and I was treated as a teacher, traditionally a respectful position in Afghanistan. We were all employed by the same NGO but the Afghan therapists were dependent on the NGO in a different way than I was. As an expatriate within the development context I was set apart. Although 'only' a development worker, and thereby on the bottom rung of the expatriate ladder, I was still in a position of power. I perceived expectations that I could access the management, where the core was largely comprised of expatriates. This management was at the top of the hierarchy and inaccessible to the therapists.

As discussed in chapter four, this had implications for the research; it also had implications for how Jenny and the therapists participated in the development project.

Power must be understood in context. Power is a natural part of interactions between humans but the understanding of it, the authority and expectations related to it, will differ in different cultural contexts, such as between high- and low power distance cultures. This has ramifications for any work where different cultures meet and people interact based on different perspectives of what power means for the roles and positions involved. If this is not understood, then when given the potential of power through the expectations placed on one's role or position, there is a risk of weaving further the hierarchical web that shapes roles and identities in both work and relationships. Being in contexts where money and power speak the loudest and where hierarchy is a given norm (and where the goal is to climb higher on the hierarchical ladder) there is an even greater need for humility and sensitivity to the power factor.

This is no simple feat. Plays of power can be deviously obscure. Every context comes with a history and every individual comes with an intricate collection of past experiences that has shaped who they are. As Jenny experienced and observed in Afghanistan, personal agendas could get in the way of the larger goal and thwart collaborative efforts – with both Afghans and expatriates. Understanding this, as part of the larger complex picture of what it means to work in another culture, or with people from another culture, is one of the aspects that are required in developing cultural reflectiveness – which we will come back to in a later chapter.

What about power plays in relation to coming to Sweden as a refugee? Regardless of what position or status a person has had before, when they flee from their country they are at the complete mercy of the authority in the new country. The new country has total control and power over the refugees – including in low PDI countries like Sweden. This means a total loss of control and power by the refugees. This loss of control can create strong anxiety and stress, even more so when the person comes from a country where the authority has all the power and wields it for its own benefit and not for the people.

For example, a study conducted by Fatumo and her colleagues (14) showed that Somali-born parents were stressed and afraid that Swedish child welfare services would perceive them as incompetent parents according to Swedish norms, and take away their children; they thought that their parenting orientation might differ from what is expected in the new country. But they also experienced a lack of understanding from the social services. Why did the Somali-born parents in that study, who came as refugees, have those fears and/or experience of the social services?

Fatumo:

From my knowledge of Somalia, the Somali government has never interfered in family issues. These were something families solved themselves. But here in Sweden the authorities intervene when it comes to what is best for the children, when it is felt that the care-givers can't do it. However, the Somali-born immigrants in the mentioned study had the experience of their government from Somalia interfering in other issues which might result in bad experiences such as imprisonment.

Another factor in the fear and the stress that the parents felt in the new country could be the loss of the collective context they knew before and the individualistic context they were in now. They expressed a feeling of loneliness caused by lack of a social network and social support. Losing their position in a group, they also lost their sense of control and power over their situation.

The power relation should thus be considered with regards to the individual's cultural, social and political position. Their state of being will be impacted by how comfortable they are in the system of practices they find themselves in, and of which they are a part. In the last example, there are different power relationships between the refugees who have fled from their countries and the authority in the new country. They have different cultural backgrounds, social resources and personal experiences which might affect the way they interact and communicate with each other and how they interpret the shared situation. This will directly impact the energy that is given or taken in the interaction.

Energy

As per the definition, energy is related to power in that power is the energy involved in moving objects. Our bodies need energy, to keep all its subsystems functioning, to live. The energy we want to talk about here, however, is the less tangible energy of social interaction. You can't see the energy but you can instinctively feel it and you can see the effects of it.

We all know the feeling that we can get from different people. Some people seem to exude energy and it spills over on others. A simple interaction with these people can leave us feeling happier and better about ourselves. We can't put our finger on why. At the other end of the spectrum there are people who with their mere presence seem to suck energy out of us. Some people gain energy from domineering over and controlling others, some people gain energy from helping others. Simply put, we have positive energy, and we have negative energy. Positive energy is constructive, negative energy is destructive. The transfer of this energy is directly dependent on context and individual. Again, we come back to why we do the things we do.

This human energy is a formidable means that we can transform to positive or to negative ends. It is a driving force that has the power to unite peoples, to create trust and a feeling of safety, to strengthen relations and build well-functioning communities. It can also be despairingly destructive and damage individuals, communities and whole systems of practices. How can we affect our own impact on others so that we produce constructive rather than destructive energy?

> Reflection:
> Think of situations where you felt that
> you could do anything and where you inspired others.
> Where did that feeling come from?

How sensitive we are to the energy given or taken by others is not constant. Sometimes we are affected by the negative energy we get from others and sometimes we can resist it. For example, Fatumo recalls two situations where her response to negative energy impacted the outcome of the interaction:

Fatumo:

One time I met a man on the street who was drunk, he swore at me "to go back home" (i.e. Somalia). I reacted and swore back, which was not a good idea because he hit me. I could have walked away from him and his verbal abuse. Instead, I absorbed his negative energy and it affected me in a destructive way leading to physical abuse. Another time a woman told me to "go back home". This time my reaction was different and I smiled and responded that I am on my way home. This made the woman calm down and she walked away.

So, even when we perceive negative energy from others, what we do with that energy is up to us, and the way we respond can lead to very different outcomes. Why do some people exude this negative or destructive energy? Is it their sense of a loss of power? Fear of that which is different? Fear of change? Fear is a powerful force that we will come back to later in this chapter.

The amount of energy we generate can have a direct impact on the way we build our relationships, the way we give agency to each other, the way we allow each other to grow and learn. Often, we can decide how we choose to respond to the energies that we are subjected to and we can learn from our responses. To do this requires the ability to take a step back, and look at what is going on. We will come back to this when we look at reflection.

Values: right and wrong

Values guide our actions. Values are not something we are born with. Values are shaped and moulded in the social and cultural circumstances in which we find ourselves and in which we grow up. Values are not set in stone.

This brings us to the real challenge in this chapter. We are not all going to share the same values. We will have different ideas about what is right and wrong. Thus, when it comes to right and wrong we come to a whole different level of complexity. Who has the right to define what is right and what is wrong? Whose practice is correct? Is there such a thing as right and wrong?

Opinions regarding right and wrong are based on long traditions of belief, power, rewards and punishments. Consider medicine as an example. There is an array of different medical practices around the world and what we said was best practice 30 years ago is not best practice now. We used to tell patients to rest when they had an injury. Now we know that too much rest can be harmful and we generally want movement as much and as quickly as possible. We have both worked in situations where we do not agree with how patients have been treated. Yet the treating medical professional fully believes s/he is in the right. Both sides can provide evidence-based arguments for their case. So, who is right? Can we base our opinion on research when research can be interpreted in many ways and scientific papers can often be found to support both sides of an argument?

The human body is intensely complex, and it lends itself to an array of different interpretations when it comes to health and wellbeing. Different cultures have different medical traditions, different explanations for why things go wrong and what should be done to treat the problem. Treating professionals will base their treatments on their understanding of the body, which is rooted in sociocultural ideals and beliefs. Spending time with different health professionals from different cultures is a great learning experience in this regard!

This is fine on an anecdotal note, but it can be very difficult in practice, when it disturbs what we believe is the best course of action. It is, of course, not limited to the field of healthcare and medicine. Our social lives are full of these challenges, where we will meet people who have strong opinions about what is right or wrong – on everything from potty training to wearing a veil. We will meet different ideas on every level, from around the coffee table at work, to the political arena.

These issues can be challenging, personally, morally, ethically and philosophically. Things are rarely black and white, and when we start exploring our ideals we may enter grey zones we didn't realise we had. Unfortunately, for a variety of reasons, we sometimes put aside our values to fulfil perceived needs, or we succumb to the views of those around us; we don't want to stand out or cause a fuss. We justify our actions in light of 'the greater good'.

An extreme example here is torture. Is it right to torture one person for the professed safety of many? Who has the power to decide this? Why is it that certain countries take the right to torture captives while condemning the torture of their own people when they are taken by 'terrorist' groups? What is the difference? Why is it considered acceptable to kill strangers in war, but a crime to kill a stranger on the street. What about bombing a wedding-party in the Middle-East, and a mass-shooting of children in a school in North America? Which gets the most attention?

There is an unspoken but clear value placed on lives depending on where these lives are from that is, at root, not only ethically and morally disturbing, but logically incomprehensible. From each side of the fence, a person's reason for doing what they do is justified based on their beliefs of what is right and wrong. One problem is that the consequent actions can contradict each other. An even deeper problem is the lack of respect and humanity toward lives of other human beings irrespective of their beliefs and values.

In our view, based on a respect for the human being, for others and for the world we live in, we do not agree with practices that in any form or way cause harm to oneself, someone else or the environment. We know, however, that there are people who have different ideas about this, or who agree, but have different definitions for what this means, or feel that there are different degrees of harm. We can thus share these base values but have different definitions of them in relation to practice. One issue that is rife in Europe is the vastly different ideas about the head covering worn by many Muslim women. This has led to harm, and to fear. The attitudes attached to this can be based on very similar beliefs and principles, but they take very different form. Two people, who share the same base value of doing no harm to others, can have radically different ideas on what this means in different practices.

For example, the first person has strong opinions about women who wear a veil, saying that it is disrespectful of women to make them cover their heads. It violates their rights. They have no issue with women being exposed wearing bikinis or underwear, on billboards, in magazines and on beaches. A second person cannot understand why women are thus publicly exposed wearing virtually nothing. They say that this is disrespectful of women. Instead, they consider women covering their head as a matter of respect and care.

Both people believe in the rights of women and both respect women. But they have very different ideas about what this means. Their definitions grow out of different world-views. Both have strong reasons and justifications for their beliefs yet they are each other's opposites. Sadly, these different understandings have led to harm.

Fatumo wears a veil and she constantly gets comments about it or questions about who has forced her to wear it.

What would her husband say if she decided to take it off; doesn't the veil impede on her freedom?

Fatumo:

Sometimes when the people realise that I work in a university as a teacher and am doing doctoral research, they ask if my husband is from the same country or if he is Swedish. These questions make me sad because people think that having a piece of cloth in your head means that you also covering your head. By asking if my husband is from Sweden, they assume both that I am not Swedish, and that a man from 'my country' would not allow me to become educated. However, I understand that this stands for their prejudices and lack of knowledge, so most of the time I try answering these questions without taking them personally.

We can grow up with others in the same city and have very different ideas about what we mean about our values. Or we can grow up in different cultures with different religions, as Jenny and Fatumo did, and share many values and beliefs. We can also have different values and ideas but still get on well and respect each other. Collaborating, living and learning together is not only about context and culture. It is not only about who we are as individual persons, nor is it even about the values and beliefs we have.

Fatumo:

I have developed my values over the years. They were not something I was born with or inherited from my family. My values have changed over time and I recognise these changes when I meet other people, families and relatives that I haven't met in years. For example, I had a discussion with a male cousin about gender issues. We were talking about politics and had different views about whether women should be allowed to be presidents or not. Our discussions became theological and it became clear that we interpreted verses from the Koran and Hadith differently. We both now live in Europe and have been influenced by the values of the countries in which we live, in my case Sweden, a country known for its gender equality (though we still have our struggles and we have more work to do!). We fully agreed that women should have the same right to education, but we differed on the issue of national leadership. By crossing borders, living and learning with people who have different ideas, I have changed my values, consciously and unconsciously.

So how do we deal with all these different ideas and opinions and beliefs? How do we avoid cultural relativism (which maintains that we cannot interfere with someone else's practice because they have their right to believe what they want)? How do we live and learn peacefully together with people who might have radically different ideas than us?

> Reflection:
> What is your core belief regarding what is right and wrong? What do you find difficult with the practices of others, and why?

The state of fear

Finally, we need to talk about fear. We are not referring to the state of fear linked to environmental catastrophe that is the topic of the book by Michael Crichton quoted earlier. Fear is a powerful force that can drive us to do any number of things. Fear can be blinding. Fear can make us do things that, in retrospect, we would not have chosen to do given more clarity of mind. Fear shuts us down. It closes us to life, to people and to ourselves.

The world appears to have become full of fear of others and fear of the unknown. Fear creates the divisions 'us' and 'them'. Sometimes the fear is not obvious; you think you are rationalising, but deep inside the fear slowly festers. What about fear of that which is different? Fear of that which we consider to be wrong? Fear of ideas that challenge our own? Fear of people who might come and compete for our jobs? These fears are very real for many people.

The fear we feel may also be irrational to others. For example, when Jenny moved to Sweden – a dream for many people – she felt considerable fear towards that which was new and unknown and strange. When she left Pakistan the experience of 'losing' so many people that she loved led to self-made barriers which prevented her from letting people get too close for fear of being hurt or alone again. But when she went to Afghanistan at the age of 24 to do a short research project, she felt no fear of going into something unknown, a place many considered dangerous. When she returned to Afghanistan to work one and a half years later, despite the growing unrest, she never once was afraid. This may appear paradoxical. Yet the fear of losing people she loved was very strong and prevented her from letting people get too close. The fear of potential injury or death in Afghanistan was never perceived as such, since Afghanistan was felt to be similar to Pakistan, which she knew well.

In essence, fear stems from self-preservation. Overcoming fear often requires that one must envision scenarios where something more important – something better – motivates you more strongly than fear, instead of dwelling on feelings of threat (personal, existential, relational, cultural, situational).

Fatumo:

Some time ago my uncle told me about the educational past of the females in our family, most of whom are highly educated now. He said it was not a coincidence but a conscious decision taken by my maternal grandfather – without fear. It was during a time when the Italian colony in Somalia provided education through the Italian church. The Somalian families were generally afraid to send their children to these schools: how can you let the power which treats you as inferior take care of your children? They were also afraid that their children would be converted to Christianity. My grandfather, who was both an Imam (a worship leader of a mosque) and a Koran teacher, decided to send all his children – both girls and boys – to school. This differed from the more common approach of other parents, who would only send the boys, or one of the boys, to school. My grandfather's decision to give the opportunity to all of his children has filtered down to his grandchildren, and it has made us who we are today. He dared to meet the unknown and to try to understand different perspectives.

We have both met and known people who fear losing control, they fear those who believe differently than themselves, they fear losing their jobs, they fear getting old. When spelled out, many fears do not make sense. As mentioned before, fear is not always logical, but it can be debilitating. It affects what we do in life and it affects how we interact with others. Ignoring fear that is there will just make things worse. Dare to face your fear, as the quote states earlier in this book.

Jenny was discussing fear of heights and climbing with a friend who had just started climbing, and how limiting this can be: knowing you are safe on a rope makes no difference at all. This friend has a fear of heights, yet he chose to persist with the climbing, trying again, slowly reaching higher, one hold at a time. Eventually he made it to the top. We can beat fear. We can, with logical thinking, reason that everything is ok, and that fear is a construction of the mind. We can overcome fear and climb to the top of the cliff.

Having said this, we know it is *not* as simple as the above analogy might suggest. In fact, it can be very difficult. Our minds are powerful things, but they are not set in stone. We can change them and overcome fear. Fear tells you that there is something in you that limits you, so do not let fear dictate how you should see and live in the world. Engaging in this change takes conscious and consistent effort. It helps to have other people with us, to be sounding boards, to create support systems, to help us see beyond our own limiting perspectives. Others can help us face and deal with our fears. Again, those with different perspectives can sometimes be the best help.

Fear, values, energy, power, forces. These mean something in relation to others. By ourselves we do not have the same need for these. So, how do we fit all this into the equation of collaboration? How can we use an understanding of all this to grow as individuals and to work together in a way that helps us all to grow and develop? That is what the next section is about.

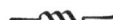

PART TWO:

Living and learning across borders

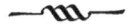

5 Participation

LEARNING IN PRACTICE

> [Participation is an] encompassing process of
> being active participants in the practices of
> social communities and constructing identities
> in relation to these communities. ...
> Such participation shapes not only what we do,
> but also who we are and how we interpret what we do.
>
> Etienne Wenger (15)

Those who have children, or spend time with children as they develop and grow, can vouch for the amazing way in which a child learns. They take on the world with vigour, they participate with all senses. They fall, they make mistakes, they get up and they try again. We watch children and recognise mannerisms that they have picked up from their parents and other close adults around them. As adults we lose some of the intensity of learning through participation. But we still do this throughout life.

This is not a theoretical, academic chapter about the intricacies of participation and learning in practice; others have written much on this (for example, see Lave and Wenger's 'situated learning' (16)). This chapter is rather a reflection on participation and learning in practice, in relation to what we have learned through reading material that others have written, through participating in a range of different contexts, through making mistakes, and through sometimes getting it right.

Participation has many sides and it is subject to a number of impacting factors. What we will consider here is participation as a key prerequisite for collaborative learning in practice, where the manner of our participation will affect how we can work and learn together.

Participation

The nature of participatory philosophy and practice is complex. It is contextual and it is dependent on the expectations of those involved. It is based on values that we hold, and on power. As a newcomer to a country, a new situation, a new job, you are dependent on others giving you agency to do things. You will also be impacted by those who enter your context as a newcomer and how you give them agency.

We have both experienced various impacting factors of participation in all the different jobs we have had. For example, Jenny's job in Afghanistan was varied and she was involved in several different professional areas. A key aspect was working with the Afghan physiotherapists to both support the development of their clinical practice and strengthen the physiotherapy department. She had great expectations of working closely with a group of senior physiotherapists and, together with them, developing the physiotherapy component. Despite knowing that there would be different attitudes owing to different backgrounds, education and cultures, she did not give enough consideration to the fact that she and the Afghan therapists might have different definitions and understandings of participation: "participation is a rich concept that means different things to different people in different settings. For some, it is a matter of principle; for others, a perspective; and for still others, an end in itself" (17). In the development project she viewed participation both as an end (increased responsibility of the supervisors = less dependency on expatriates) and a means (facilitating improvement of their clinical practice that was suited to the Afghan therapists' context). As the development project progressed she perceived that she and the therapists had different expectations each other's roles. This had direct implications for their participation.

Jenny:

I came with a perspective of striving towards equal participation and responsibility in the project. I entered a hierarchical context where I was met by expectations of bringing new techniques, new knowledge and skills. Although I was young, I felt that I was expected to be the expert, with my Western education and degree. It was explained to me, and I experienced in practice, that patients had a greater belief in treatment suggested or given by an expatriate physiotherapist.

Although I started as a volunteer (and thereby on the lowest rank amongst the expatriates), I was treated as an advisor. I was part of the Technical Support Unit for the programme, based in the central management office in Kabul. Together with the Afghan Physiotherapy Officer I held a position of responsibility in the physiotherapy component. I was expected to solve problems and lobby for the therapists as well as teach and supervise. All of this led to a particular place in the hierarchy. On the other hand, my younger age and unmarried status demanded less respect compared with older colleagues, which – with my hope of more horizontal collaboration – was felt to be an asset.

The experiences from this research impressed upon me the importance of critically reflecting over one's own role and position in participating in and researching others' practice. It is not enough to consider the issues beforehand or afterwards, rather a constant reflection must be done when in the field. One's attitude and cultural sensitivity lies at the heart of being able to conduct both research and development work in an ethical manner.

As people, we generally want to be included, to feel that we belong to a group or community, that we have the space and the means to participate in a practice. We talk about the importance of diversity, of integration, but what do we really mean by this? Do we want people from different groups, ideologies, cultures or religions to coexist? Do we want people to participate in society on equal terms? If so, we have some work to do.

Fatumo:

In my experience, people talk about migrants, how they do not want to be integrated in the society or how they should be integrated. There is less talk of inclusion or how we can support and enable people to be included in the society. When I came to Sweden and got my permit, the first move I did to be included in my new home was to learn the language. Then I started to look for work. Unfortunately, with every job I applied for I got the same comments "do you have any experience?" Every time I replied: "I have cleaned my whole life, and that is experience". But that was not good enough. How could I get any experience when I was never given the chance? It was not easy to overcome these barriers, but I did. Step by step I got a profession: I become a nurse. This facilitated entering the labour market. It was a struggle from my side, to not give up and see every challenge as a part of pursuing my dream. With the support of others, I was able to continue on my path of development and enter doctoral studies.

Now, I feel included most of the time at my work, but that has not always been the case. It has been, and it still is, tough to be in academia. I have struggled to become a part of the academic world. I was lucky to have people who believed in me and they changed others belief in me. My participation in academia thus depends on having people who include me and invite me to be a part of it, people who act as mentors and role models, who try to give me agency and who advocate for me. This is the conclusion I made several years ago: "I was in the right place, at the right time and met the right people".

When you are a newcomer in a country you need the people in the new system to give you opportunities and the agency to participate. Participation in this regard should not have to come down to chance, about meeting the right people at the right time and place.

In terms of the experiences described, we both struggled with participation, but for different reasons. We both wanted to participate in the new contexts we were in, we were both dependent on the agency given to us from the people around us. But the reasons for our challenges of participation were very different, due to who we were perceived to be in relation to the new context. We have both experienced, and experience, what it means to be treated in a way that does not correlate with how we feel about ourselves, based on the tone of our skin, the clothes we wear, even the hairstyle we chose.

In terms of the Swedish context, we hear talk about people who are immigrants, unemployed etc. not wanting to participate or contribute to society. We hear disgruntled comments about them just "taking grants from the government and living off our taxes". Crime is more easily blamed on 'the others'. But is this true? How do we know? Have we asked those individuals what they want or how they can participate? Importantly, do we give them the chance and opportunity to participate?

Time and time again it seems that as a group, we see segregation but don't look for what causes it, we don't look for the roots. We think that people generally have a desire to belong to something, to participate. Participation means having a voice and making decisions together with other people. But instead of allowing this, we think on behalf of other people, based on what we think they want, which stems from our understanding of the world, and of what we think is right and wrong.

> Reflection:
> How does it feel when someone makes a decision for you without asking you what you want? When was the last time you had an opinion about what others should be doing without checking about their opinion on the matter?

Academia and research are not exempt from this in our experience. When conducting research on immigrant/ethnic minorities or people from other cultures, how much of this is done with a true representation of them in the actual research? When there is no participation of the people being researched, we may produce research with cultural stereotyping and there is a risk of the research being self-serving. If we involve individuals who have a similar background to the people being studied it often appears they are used more as assistants or informants, to recruit and collect data etc. The analysis is done by those who are not of the same group and is thus interpreted from perspectives that might be very different from the group being studied.

On the news, we can sometimes see people who claim they are expert on a group of people or ethnic minority, and speak on their behalf. But how often do these 'experts' speak the language of the people they claim to know so well? By whose definition are they experts and to what extent? Can Jenny claim that she is expert on Pakistani, Afghani or Emirati people, just because she spent years in their countries? Can Fatumo claim she is an expert on Ethiopian or Kenyan people? Can we claim to be experts on Swedes? Can we ever become experts on others?

Development work suffers from the same problem. Participatory approaches in development work are a growing trend, yet this does not annul the risk of Western concepts of development directing the participation or the issue of who has power.

For example, in employing a participatory approach in the development project and her research, Jenny did not fully comprehend the complexities of what such work entails as part of the development context. She recalls feeling uncomfortable with conducting research in Afghanistan, concerned that she would be talking about the physiotherapists. This was an underlying reason for the participatory nature of the research approach she chose. Her manner of participation was central, yet she was less critical of this when in the field. Jenny looks back and can see how naïve she was. She discovered the importance of self-critical reflection over her own manner of participation (18). She learned in practice that participation is deeply linked to the factors discussed in the previous section, where expectations have roots in deeper ideals and are dependent on power. She thus experienced the value of participation for learning in practice.

Reflection:
Think about a situation in your life where you have participated in a new context.
How did you engage in the new practice?

How did others respond to you?
Then think about a situation
where new people have come into your context.
How did you engage with them?
How did you allow/not allow them to participate?

Learning in practice

If we let it, participation can lead to fabulous learning. Through actively engaging with the people and practices around us we can learn a lot about ourselves, about others, about how things (techniques, apparatus, etc) work in practice, far beyond what we read in books or learn from research, university studies and courses. With participation in this respect, we don't mean simply being in a context and doing the work.

We are social beings and we learn from each other. Some of this happens automatically. We unconsciously pick up unspoken social rules, mannerisms and ways of speaking, simply by being around other people. By nature, some do this more, some less. Consider language and mannerisms of communication. Fatumo tends to change expressions, intonations and gestures whenever she changes languages from Swedish to Somali or Arabic:

Fatumo:

I remember when I returned to Somalia for the first time after I had been in Sweden for 19 years. Speaking with staff at the Berbera airport, I started to speak a little louder than I did when I spoke in Swedish. My Swedish colleagues who were with me were surprised by my manner and thought I was yelling and arguing with the staff. I was so surprised how I could switch ways of speaking so easily.

Similarly, Jenny's English changes when she is in a context with more British English speakers or with more American

English speakers. Her mannerisms also change depending on the social context she is in. She does this unconsciously but she notices the difference in the way she speaks when she is, for example, in Sweden or the UK or France.

Although we both have the habit of altering our ways of communicating depending on the context, this is not the case with everyone. Different people have different levels of adjusting and picking up local ways of being and doing things. Some people have an uncanny and enviable ability to pick up other languages and social habits seemingly without trying; others can spend years in one place and maintain their dialect and mannerisms, or struggle to learn the new language.

Then there are other aspects of learning that do not happen without more conscious effort. There is also the matter of our interest in learning, and in the agency given to us to participate in a manner that enables learning. If we enter something new and we feel fear or suspicion, how well will we learn the new social and cultural codes? With attitudes such as this, one may use that which is new and different to reinforce old ideas and beliefs rather than learn new nuances and perspectives.

Jenny and Fatumo have both been in situations like this. Spending time with other people doesn't mean we will learn from them. Traveling does not automatically mean we will have a better understanding of the world. So how do we encourage constructive, balanced learning in practice that can enable us to learn from each other and to live together respectfully and peacefully? This is not an easy thing at all. We will come back to this later in the book.

There is another dimension to learning in practice. As we engage in a practice or context and learn together with others, we will have an impact on the context. We will have an impact on the culture. Looking at our Swedish context with its various subcultures (is there one Swedish culture?), we can see how it has changed through the years as the demographic of Sweden has changed. These changes are apparent in how we greet each other, in the language, in the groceries available in stores, in what is portrayed in movies and on television.

This has always been happening. What we know at a certain point in time as a specific culture was not the same 20, 100 or 300 years ago. The nature of our cultural world is that these cultures are changing. The cultures of the Americas before Columbus were very different to those which developed after Europeans arrived. The culture of the United States of America today is what it is because of all the different people from all over the world, who have contributed to make it what it is. In Europe, we also have much influence from the rest of the world due to the years of colonisation. A few years ago Jenny read an old book about bread from an English author where it was stated that curry was the quintessential British spice. Although the mix 'curry powder' is a Western creation, the spices that make up the curry powder are not native to the British Isles; they come from South Asia. Examples such as this are numerous.

Our countries have always been changing, so why is there such fear about this? Where does the nationalistic attitude come from that is so resistant to new people coming into our countries? Why view them with such contempt and fear instead of curiosity and the potential for learning all kinds of new and exciting things? We seem to have forgotten where we are from in a historical sense. We do not own the land. (And if we think we do own it, why do we not make more of an effort to take care of it rather than destroy it the way we seem to be very successfully doing at the moment?)

We have created borders in an effort to organise ourselves. This is fine: organisation is helpful. But if we continue hardening these borders, speaking ill of others, treating them badly, we are heading down a destructive path. To every action there is an equal and opposite reaction. This basic physics principle is something we learned in school. But when it comes to life we don't appear to realise that treating others badly can start a negative chain reaction. What does treating refugees badly do to them? Many have paid a huge price to leave their countries, financially, emotionally and physically. Lives have been lost. Children have experienced things that no-one should have to experience. These people may become part of new contexts and cultures in the new country. They can bring new things to their new systems of practice. But if they are treated with suspicion and are kept at a distance, why be surprised if there are repercussions? When young men are angry and do hurtful things? We all have parts to play in the ways our societies work. The Golden Rule suits very well here: 'Do to others what you would have them do to you'.

How can we turn our and others' participation in practice into positive and constructive learning that enables us to live together respectfully? What have we learned through our different experiences of moving to new places, starting new jobs, working in new and different cultural systems and practices, of doing research, of working with people to try to help their pain?

We can read as many books as we want or take as many courses as we want, but if we don't actively engage in critically reflecting over our manner of participation, over what we are told or how we are treated in relation to the world we are experiencing and living in, then we will not 'learn' from our experiences. We might have an idea nestled somewhere in our brain, but that idea may not be relevant in relation to others or to the situation or context we are in. It can become destructive when we base our actions only on our own understanding of the world.

> Reflection:
> Can you recall situations where you participated in a practie in a positive way? What were your driving forces? How did you engage people so they you could learn from each other? Can you think of situations where you have acted on your own ideas without discussing them with others? Have there been consequences to this?

Many people have written much more eloquently and in depth on this topic and we do not venture to compete with that. We will offer our own version of support for how to enhance learning in practice, and that version will be presented in two later chapters in relation to reflection. This act of reflection requires communicative reflection (19) with others. So let's first take a look at communication.

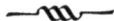

6 communication

THE ART OF LISTENING AND SPEAKING

> If the person you are talking to doesn't appear to be listening, be patient. It may simply be that he has a small piece of fluff in his ear.
>
> Winnie the Pooh

Jenny:

In Pakistan in the last couple of decades of the twentieth century we did not have the Internet or mobile phones. We had a black-and-white TV that showed five minutes of cartoons in the afternoon. I wrote my first essay on a computer in the final year of high school. We had to book phone-calls to Sweden through an operator, and then we had three precious crackling minutes to split between the six of us. We recorded cassette tapes that we sent back and forth between Sweden and Pakistan. We wrote letters, carefully lovingly penned for the people far from us.

Fatumo:

After I left Somalia and came to Nairobi I had to travel to Mombasa for 9 hours just to call my family on a satellite phone. It was the only means of communication to families in Somalia at the time, to let them know that we were okay. There was no guarantee that you would get through. You had to call and make an appointment for the following day, and then success depended on the operator staff being able to find your family. The operator place we called from was not fancy, it was a satellite phone placed on a boat. It was similar when I came to Sweden. This time I didn't have to use a satellite phone, but it involved the same procedure of calling to make an appointment to call your family the next Saturday or Sunday depending on when they found your family.

Today the Internet spans the world. When we are away from our family and friends we communicate directly and instantly with them through email, whatsapp, Skype etc. Jenny receives little videos of her nieces' antics, and can thus follow them as they grow and develop, even when thousands of kilometres away. When she worked in Afghanistan, mobiles were standard. There was no landline as the development process had skipped straight to the mobile. Even remote villages boasted TV antennas and satellite dishes from the brown earthen rooftops. In short, we and our contemporaries now have opportunities to communicate that our grandparents would never have dreamed of when they were our age.

Yet with all this communications technology literally at our fingertips, are we better at communicating? Has this enabled us to cross barriers (virtual and real) or are we actually enhancing them? It seems that, more and more, we hide behind the safety and efficacy of a text rather than a phone call. We may communicate more but are we actually connecting less? Social media has had a huge impact on the spreading of information, ideas and opinions. It has a huge impact on how we view ourselves and how we develop our world-view. At an individual level there appears to be a tendency to say things through social media without reflecting much on the words being written. Has this social media (where we don't need the physical interaction of face-to-face communication) affected our filter of empathy?

Communication is thus no guarantee for dialogue; it can be quite the opposite. We can communicate with each other without feeling that we are participating or having any affinity with each other. So, let's look more at this. We will first discuss the spoken dialogue, the words we share when we communicate, and then the unspoken component of communication and the impact of culture.

The spoken word

To communicate we need a shared repertoire of signs and signals that hold shared meanings. Partly we do this with words. (We will talk about the spoken word although this also includes the signed words of sign language.) Living with people that come from different countries and people groups means living with people who may have a different repertoire of signals compared to your own. We have different languages and this naturally entails challenges, but that is not what we will consider here. What we wish to highlight is how we react to how someone uses language – in other words, the meaning we attach to what someone says.

On a course with people from many different countries Jenny met a German-speaking woman. She was gentle and quiet and didn't actively participate in the discussions. After a couple of days Jenny was chatting with her and they started talking about languages. This lady said she felt like an outsider and that she was not able to be herself. Normally she was a very chatty and outgoing person but because she was not very comfortable with speaking English she became someone that she did not recognise. She was concerned that people got the wrong impression about her.

When we meet new people we make an unconscious assessment of them. We create an idea in our mind about what they are like. When we meet people from contexts, countries or cultures other than our own, we do the same thing. The problem with this is that these people will most likely have a different language as well as a different manner of communicating (which we will come back to later). They may not be able to participate in a practice or social group the way they would like, yet we judge them on how they participate.

> Reflection:
> Think about situations in your daily life
> where you interact with people who
> come from other
> countries or cultures than your own.
> How do you view them?
> Have you been in situations where you have not
> shared the same language or means to communicate
> as everyone else and have felt excluded?
> How did this make you feel?
> Could you or the people you interacted with,
> have done differently?

Communication is a social act. We don't only express our views; we also express who we are. The spoken word is only one aspect. We can say one thing while our whole body language says something quite different. We can learn a new language but we also need to learn the unspoken aspect of communication.

The art of communication

In the early days of the telephone one could say that necessity demanded dialogue, with a balance between listening and speaking. The delay in the conversation meant that one had to pause and listen carefully to what the person on the other end was saying. Today we communicate largely with e-mail, texts/sms, various messaging apps and other similar written messages. In these forms of communication, the art of listening (and speaking) is not practiced. (Not to mention the art of writing, but that is a discussion for another time!)

What does this mean? Artful communication is the balanced combination of listening and speaking, each having an array of nuances. Artful communication takes into account the context we are in and the scope for variation that may exist and of which we weren't previously aware. You can never predict where it will take you.

Communicating artfully does not mean agreeing on everything or coming to a consensus. We don't have to agree, and that need not be the aim. We do, however, need to learn to co-exist respectfully, which entails communicating respectfully. This brings us to another challenge: it takes two (at least) to communicate artfully. If we do not agree on something, and only one person seeks to understand the other, then how do we move forward? What if we feel that we have been wronged or slighted in some way? What, and how, do we communicate then?

There are many layers and angles to this and there is no easy format to follow. Each situation will have its own myriad social/personal conditions and consequences, and in each situation we will need to find a unique path to a solution. We will not always get answers in the end, but it is the process of striving to find an answer that can lead us forward. This is the art. To strive to listen beyond the words being said and listen to the words in context. We will come back to this in the next chapter in relation to how we as individuals engage together with others and how we try to learn from situations that 'push our buttons' or leave us feeling challenged or in some way affected.

As we engage more and more with each other and learn not to fear that which is different, or to fear our own shortcomings, it can become easier to communicate well. In this respect, it helps to consider the way we communicate and the part context plays. Much of how we communicate is influenced by culture and the manner of communication used when we were growing up.

Communication and culture

When we talk to people from other cultures it may be that things are not as we initially perceive them to be. If someone doesn't respond the way you are used to, it probably is not that they have some fluff in their ear (as suggested by Winnie the Pooh), but that they have a different manner of communicating. It could be the eye contact. If could be the delay in answering. It could be a more direct or a more roundabout reply than you are accustomed to. Let's consider eye contact as an example.

In Sweden, you are expected to keep eye contact with the person you are talking to, whether it be a man or woman. If you avoid eye contact it may appear that you are hiding something, or perhaps you are very shy. In other countries, such as Somalia, avoiding eye contact means respecting the other person. But this does not mean that all Somali people perceive it so. Even here, there are more things to consider such as specific context, situation, power, etc. Each situation depends on the interplay between ourselves and the person we are communicating with.

Another common example relates to how we communicate in situations of conflict. How conflicts were solved when we were children will often shape how we approach difficult situations as adults. How you were treated as a child and what communication practices you grew up with, may dictate your ability to handle criticism or praise. It may dictate the manner in which you speak with others. Trying to understand this can be very helpful in understanding how people respond and act when communicating in 'conflict' situations.

> Reflection:
> How did your family handle conflicts when you were growing up? How were problems communicated? Has this had an impact on how you communicate in challenging situations?

There are also cultural variations in how we express ourselves verbally. It is not only the actual words that have meaning, but also who said the words to whom, the relationships involved, where they were said, what has been said previously etc. The contextual/personal factors and the forces of human interaction (chapters 2-4) all have an impact on communication. There are cultural variations when people from different cultures communicate. The variations lie in how we interpret the underlying meaning of the words that are said and how they are said. Hall has divided these variations into *low-context* (LC) and *high-context* (HC) communication (20).

LC communication is characterised by information being given in explicit ways; nothing is left unsaid and the information might be repeated to ensure that the other person has understood and to increase the credibility of what is said. Silence and pauses in the communication can be perceived as a lack of interest or disagreement. HC communication is characterised by information which is embedded in the physical context, or internalised in the person. Much of the message is left unspoken and is more likely to be read 'between the lines'. Over-emphasis is perceived as confusion on the part of the person speaking.

A low-context communication style is more prevalent in Sweden and other Nordic countries, for example, and high-context communication is common in Somalia and other countries in Africa and Asia. There are also variations within these countries, and there is no such thing as one absolute form of communication in each place, but there are tendencies that stand out. Fatumo grew up in an HC communication country and then moved to a LC communication country. She recalls an example of where she – who has both LC and HC communication styles (even if she tends more towards HC) – had difficulty in understanding a person with a HC communication style:

Fatumo:

I went to see a neighbour, who is from Somalia, to help her with something for just a few minutes. While we were talking, I said something like "I haven't eaten all day". The next minute I had food in front of me. I was using LC communication while my neighbour interpreted my words from a HC communication perspective. In other words, her interpretation of what I said was "I am hungry and want to eat something". We laughed about this some years later when I explained our little misunderstanding.

I've also experienced LC and HC communication differences at work. Sometimes I get irritated when some of my colleagues repeat the same information several times as if I were unable to understand them the first time. But then I remind myself that we have different ways of communicating. For example, one colleague wanted to be explicit with her communication and make sure that everything was clear, using LC communication. I, on the other hand, used my HC communication style. I understood the information the first time and I also read between the lines of what she was saying. It could also be that I was not using the body language that she was familiar with and so she could not see from my expression or body language that I understood her.

Jenny also recalls numerous situations in Afghanistan and the UAE where she and the other person in the interaction had different modes of communication (LC and HC), which led to misunderstandings and misinterpretations. The important thing to remember is that these differences in communication style are never static and there are myriad other factors involved (such as the various forces affecting us, discussed in chapter 4). With our experiences from different contexts, we have both learned to communicate with HC and LC styles. We can switch between them, although this is not always entirely straightforward, depending on the situation and context at hand. There are more things that play a part. One very important dimension to communication is the unspoken, non-verbal aspect.

Body language

Anyone who has travelled and been observant of other ways of being will likely have noticed the different mannerisms and actions that people use in their conversations, particularly when emphasising or illustrating a point they are making. This adds colour and life to a conversation. For some, face-to-face communication is not done through words at all but through the intricate hand-dance of sign language.

Whether we speak with our mouths and listen with our ears, or speak with our hands and listen with our eyes, communicating in person involves a repertoire of signals of the body that are not involved when using only written forms of communication. In addition to words we have a whole array of non-spoken messages being transferred, by how we stand, the expressions on our faces and how we use our hands. The same words can be given completely different meanings depending on this non-spoken communication. When we listen, the way we listen in terms of eye contact or posture can give away whether we are interested by what is being said. We speak and we listen with our whole bodies.

How we phrase our words, how we combine our spoken and non-spoken communication, is intricately dependent on context, who we are in relation to the other person, what system of practices we have grown up in, and what the expectations are in the dialogue. As mentioned before, this is tightly linked to culture. What is inviting in one culture can be offensive in another and vice versa. This non-verbal communication can be harder to learn if we are not observant and reflective about what we are doing, what others are doing, and how they react towards us.

Growing up in Pakistan, Jenny learned the manner of communication that was expected between men and women in Pakistani systems of practices. This was very useful when she was in Afghanistan as she engaged with her Afghan colleagues. She recalls being asked about the manner of acting and communicating of some Western colleagues who – unknowingly – made cultural mistakes in their actions and communications that would have been offensive coming from an Afghan. Conversely, her experiences from Pakistan did not help her in her communication in Sweden, especially with men: when she moved back to Sweden she found communication and interaction with men much harder than with women. She did not know what social codes applied, how to differentiate between the unspoken messages of friendly interest and romantic interest. She had to learn these, through trial and error, as she engaged more and more with people in Sweden and other European countries.

When Fatumo came to Sweden and learned Swedish, she learned the non-verbal communication along with the spoken Swedish language.

Fatumo:

I don't know how this happened. I have realised I don't use the same gestures now as when I was in Somalia. Today, I automatically switch communication habits when I travel between Sweden and Somalia. However, this is not completely fluent, and through these situations I realise how much I have changed. There have been situations where I felt offended when someone used a form of non-verbal communication which to me seemed inappropriate. For example, I recall one time when I was working in a hospital in Sweden where the doctor in charge wanted to ask me a question and he pointed at me with his finger. This made me so angry, because for me it was like calling to an animal/dog, and I pretended I didn't see him until he called me by my name. This also makes me wonder: how many people I have inadvertently offended?

Another aspect of non-verbal communication is the physical space we inhabit when we are communicating with other people, i.e. personal space. Space in this respect refers to the distance between individuals when they interact with each other. All communication takes place in the context of distance. Social rules concerning personal distance differ from one culture to another and from one individual to another. We have our own personal distance according to our own territorial behaviour i.e. feelings or attitude toward our own personal space. When we interact with people we unconsciously choose a distance to that person depending on our relationship to that person. For example, a conversation between two Swedish people takes place at a longer distance than between individuals from Somalia who stand much closer while talking.

Fatumo:

A couple of years ago, I met a woman in a hair salon where we were both waiting for our turn. We talked about family and life. The next day I met her again in a bus station outside my apartment. She approached me and greeted me, and she was so close to me that I took a step backward (unconsciously) and she took one forward. I continued to move backwards and she continued to come closer. Then I stopped and thought: why was I doing that? What did my reactions stand for? Even though I was used to having less personal space with the people I interact with back in Somalia, I still reacted towards this perceived intrusion on my personal space. I do not remember when I made such change and started needing more personal space.

Smells and odours also have a powerful impact in our communication. With smells and odours, we send signals to others, and these can stimulate attraction or revulsion. What smells socially acceptable, 'good' or 'bad', depends on cultural traditions and perceptions about various smells and odours. We grow up being taught that certain smells are ok, others are not. Some smells are encouraged, others are not. We unconsciously judge others based on how they smell to us. Smells link to our memories, and certain smells and odours can remind us of previous experiences, either pleasant or unpleasant. Sometimes they just leave us with a specific feeling. Although there are cultural perceptions about certain smells (such as body odour, perfume, garlic etc.), our idea of what smells good is not necessarily the same as that of other people in the same culture or context.

Fatumo was giving a lecture about cultural encounters to health professionals in Sweden who in their daily work meet patients from different countries. She was asked why some Somali women smell so differently, with strong odours.

Fatumo:

I didn't understand what the question had to do with meeting patients. I said perhaps it was related to incense that Somali women sometimes use to freshen up the home. In an effort to really explain this, the next day I brought the incense for them to smell. I was disappointed by their response: they were not satisfied and said it was worse, it was stronger and smelled bad. This made me sad and I told them, maybe they think you smell different too!

We haven't read much about how smells relate to culture and communication, but we have experienced it. The most important thing to remember is that the way you see or smell things is not the only 'normal' or 'right' way, and others might just as well perceive your way of seeing/smelling as being awkward or odd. We will talk more in the next chapter about how what we perceive with our senses is very much an interpretation from our body. Things are often not what they initially appear to be and will appear differently to different people.

> Reflection:
> In relation to communication with others,
> how do 'not making eye contact', 'making waving gestures',
> 'standing close to another person', 'smells and odours'
> impact you, and what might they mean to another person?

Body language and non-verbal communication is intricately linked to our being-states (as discussed in chapter 3), to the context we are in and to who else is in that context (chapter 2), what their relationship is with us, and what forces are at play in our collaboration (chapter 4). The challenge when living and working together with people who have grown up in different systems of practices is that we can have very different ways of conveying our message and different ways of interpreting the messages coming in. A first step is to become aware of this and the impact it has. One way to start this process is to tell stories.

Telling stories

Part of being human is to tell stories. Through the ages and all over the world, people have told stories; stories to entertain, to educate, and to pass on morals and ethics from one generation to the next. We all have our own personal stories, and how we tell our stories says much about who we are.

Stories not only pass on an idea or a way of thinking, we also create identities with our stories. We convey hidden beliefs and values in the way we tell our stories. We want to relate the person telling stories to our own experience. Through sharing our stories, we start building a relationship, even if only briefly and in passing. We tell various stories in this book drawn from our experience. We tell stories about the body and how it works. We hope that these stories can help illustrate and inspire your stories. You may read different things into the stories that we tell than what we intended. You may not agree with all the points we have made. Perhaps you will recognise aspects of your life in our stories. Whatever your reaction is, it stems from what you have experienced and the beliefs you hold in relation to these. This is your interpretation, that you make based on your being-state and worldview.

When you hear a story you create an image in your mind based on what you know. If you have grown up in a country where it never snows, your only images of this are from movies or pictures. If you then hear someone tell a story about their holiday in the north of Sweden in the middle of winter, your interpretation of that story will be different from someone who has done a similar trip or lives in a country where snow is common. How you hear and visualise the story depends on what you have experienced before and your ability to see things from different perspectives. The story you hear is not necessarily the same as the one intended by the story teller.

We also change the way we tell our stories depending on who is listening and what our relationship is with that person. Issues such as power, fear and agency will all impact how a story is told and how it is received. When we listen to others' stories we may or may not let them change us. We may laugh. We may feel encouraged or strengthened. We may feel threatened. We may want to retaliate or defend ourselves. But however we may feel, it's not only about us; we need to learn to listen to each other's stories without judging, retaliating, or defending ourselves. The challenge is to listen without the aim of taking something for ourselves or pushing our own agenda but simply to listen to the story being told.

When stories make us feel good about ourselves this is easy. When stories challenge us it is much harder. But here is where it gets interesting. This is where we have the potential to learn and grow. It is about how we communicate together.

Communicative reflection

As has already been mentioned, it is the dialogue with others that can help us develop our own ideas and ways of thinking. We have previously talked about communicative reflection which is "the dialogical reflection over experiences based on a mutual interest of gaining a better understanding of what has been experienced" (21). Through communicative reflection we can explore the reasons for why we do what we do. We can learn about different ways of communicating. This brings us to the next chapter. What do we mean by reflection? How can we develop our skills of reflection so as to enhance our manner of participation and communication and, ultimately, our collaboration?

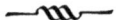

7 reflection

THE ART OF SEEING AND FEELING

> Do you have the patience to wait till
> your mud settles and the water is clear?
> Lao Tzu

Reflection has come up as a central part of how we learn in practice and of how we understand each other. Reflection is a central component of trying to understand what can be causing the pain or dysfunction with clients. Reflection is a key part of trying to understand ourselves, our actions and intentions and, based on this, we can endeavour to understand the actions and intentions of others.

We, Fatumo and Jenny, believe reflection is an essential part of what makes us who we are as thinking, learning human beings. In this book, we work from the following definition of reflection: *"a cognitive and affective process or activity that a) requires active engagement on the part of the individual; b) is triggered by an unusual or perplexing situation or experience; c) involves examining one's own responses, beliefs, and premises in light of the situation at hand; and d) results in integration of the new understanding into one's experience"* (22).

Simply put, reflection is a structured, conscious, analytic thinking process that leads to greater understanding or knowledge, leaving us in a different state than we were before. It is a continual process that helps us to grow and develop, both as individuals and professionals, and it requires active effort. Critical reflection is essentially the same, but the critically analytic process is directed towards oneself, one's experiences, actions, reactions, beliefs and interactions with others: *"Reflection enables us to correct distortions in our beliefs and errors in problem solving. Critical reflection involves a critique of the presuppositions on which our beliefs have been built"* (23). This is all fairly complex and elaborate to get one's head around, so let's take a closer look at reflection.

Reflection and refraction

The word 'reflection' comes from Latin and means 'to bend back'. When light is reflected onto a shiny surface it is 'bent back', essentially the same as it was. Reflection of light is a crucial part of transferring signals that enable the brain to create the represented image of what is 'seen'. Light can only be seen when it is reflected off a surface, and it is the reflection of light on surfaces that enables us to see the objects and colours around us.

This is a fascinating process. After being reflected off a surface, the reflected light rays first pass through the cornea and lens of the eye, where they are refracted and focused on the retina. This reflection and refraction of light onto the retina of the eye triggers a series of complex electrical signals that get passed to the brain which then makes an interpretation and tells us what we see. Similarly, reflection, as used in this book, is essentially the processing of an event or experience to enable us to 'see' what happened. How accurately can we 'see' and understand what was going on? What was impacted? This is where refraction becomes of interest.

Light travels in a straight line. If it does not reflect off a surface but passes through it (in passing from air to water for example), then refraction occurs. With refraction, light is partially bent or deflected as it passes from one medium into another. The degree of refraction depends on the medium it is passing through. So, after refraction, the direction of the line of light has changed. In the eye, this refraction occurs in the cornea and the lens and refraction enables the light to be focused on the retina so that the signals can then be sent to the brain. Without refraction there would be no perceived image in the brain.

Based on this understanding, we will also use refraction in our discussion of living and learning together. Reflection enables light to be passed to the eyes and without this we wouldn't even be aware of what was around us. But without refraction, no light would be focused on the retina and no signals would be transmitted to the brain. Thus, we would like to suggest that refraction is analogous to our critical reflection process, in particular communicative reflection. When we discuss with others what we have seen, we often get different perspectives that may or may not give us new insight and understanding, and thus slightly change the angle of our thoughts, compared to before.

There are other factors to consider related to this notion of refraction in relation to communicative reflection. We discussed world-view earlier. Our worldview will impact how we interpret the events around us. Our worldview can be likened to our eye lenses. Firstly, we develop our worldview based on how we 'see' the world – and how and what we see is based on our experiences and beliefs. Secondly, our worldview is like the lens in that this is the medium through which our experiences are filtered and focused. Also, refraction will change depending on the thickness of the lens in the eye. The condition of these lenses is partly dependent on genetic factors and age, but it will change depending on how we use them.

For example, if we spend most of our time staring at a screen, the muscles of the lens must work harder to keep the lens thicker and enable it to focus the light. Eventually the function of these muscles gets affected and we can develop short-sightedness. In the same way our worldview is dependent on how we engage with others around us. For example, if we don't engage in communicative reflection with others – in particular those who have different ideas to us – we run the risk of becoming more rigid and set in our thinking and less able to appreciate the depth and colours in the world that are beyond the view of our short-sightedness.

Having considered the way light enables signals to be passed to the brain, the next thing to consider is the role of the brain. We think we see the same thing, but seeing is an interpretation of our brains, and our brains are as different as we are as individuals.

Brain power

We see with our brain – literally. The interpretation of the electrical signals coming from the eyes to the brain is incredibly complex and dependent on a huge array of different factors which are beyond the scope of this book. But let's consider a couple things.

Our brains are fantastically plastic. Just as plastic can be moulded into different shapes, plasticity in the brain means it can change, develop, and take on new and different roles depending on the needs of the body. Our brains develop based on how they are used, depending on what signals are coming in, what our state of being is and what context we are in. Our brains have developed very much dependent on how they were stimulated as young children. They then continue changing and developing based on how we use them as adults.

Some people are colour blind. They will see a green flower when, in fact, the flower is red. But for that person, the flower is green. We can only see the world through our own eyes and we think that what we see is real. But what we see is interpreted by a brain that is not identical to anyone else's brain. Building on the above analogy, when we experience something, we filter the experience through our respective worldview lenses and filters which we have developed throughout life, and we interpret the signals coming in based on what we know of the world. Based on our experiences our interpretation of signals will change and impact what and how we see things. How would we know that we are colour blind or if what we see is what others see? The only way to find out is to talk to others and discuss what they are seeing.

Many of you will have seen optical illusions, images that play with what we see. We think we know what we see, and then our focus changes, and suddenly we see something different. So, what are we seeing? Whose version of what is seen is 'right'? If we consider what we said in an earlier chapter regarding how we communicate based on how we see things, it makes a considerable difference if we recognise that we might see different things, depending on who is doing the observing, in the same situation.

This is one of the cornerstones of reflection in relation to what we know and believe. We need to talk to others based on the understanding that we may or may not be basing what we say on a (sometimes radical) different understanding of what has occurred. If we have this shared attitude then discussing our experiences and sharing ideas and perspectives can help us develop our thinking, our understanding of each other, and show us where we might have gaps in our perspective. It can help us develop as people.

We need to want to do this. Just as we need to make an active effort to change movement behaviours (such as taking breaks from staring at the screen!), we need to want to understand what we are seeing and experiencing. We need to want to try to see things from another's perspective. We need to want to listen. All of this is taken into consideration in the basic reflection format that we will come to later in this chapter. Before we look at this format we want to make some observations about a couple other things that play into how we see and perceive things.

Gut feeling and heart ache

Most of us view the brain as the control centre of the body that sends out signals telling the body what to do and processes input coming from the body (such as from the eyes). But this is a very simplified representation of what our amazing bodies actually do and how they work (and so much of this we still don't understand!). How aware are you of the different systems involved in how your complex body system is running, or of how you feel and react?

You know that strange sensation deep in your abdomen, like something is clenching, or fluttering, or sinking, depending on the associated situation? And what about the old saying, follow your heart? Have you felt that tangible pain in your chest, in the heart area, when you have gone through grief or pain? Literally, heartache. These are real. And they affect how we feel.

Our gut is a highly complex organ. It is central to our immune system and it has more nerve cells than the peripheral nervous system. The gut supplies the brain with very important information about the inner state of the body. The inner state of our body has a direct impact on how we feel. Stress and depression are not just emotional responses, they are chemical actions taking place in our bodies. If we are upset, feel threatened or stressed, this is going to impact messages going between the gut and the brain. It appears that the state of the gut directly impacts our emotional state and whether we feel motivated or depressed. Our mental state is going to impact other signals coming in to the brain, for example, how we perceive our experiences, other people, and ourselves in relation to them.

When it comes to the heart and feeling, this is a field less explored. But in the same way that the gut has more of a function than simply digesting our food, the heart does more than just send blood around our body. The heart is constantly in communication with the brain and with the rest of the body, and alters its action based on the information coming in. The heart is thus a perceptive organ, and can pick up changes in the state of the body.

What signals we pick up from people and the world around us, what we feel, feeds into what we do. What we do and how we act on depends on whether we stop and consider what is going on, or if we react 'without thinking'. Which brings us back to reflection.

Reflection is the analytical thinking process described previously. This happens in the brain, but the process clearly has more components to it. If what is going on in the gut and the heart impacts what is going on in the brain, and what is going on in the brain impacts how we engage with the people around us, then we realise that reflection is not merely a matter of the mind.

Think about this: apart from the actual physiological impact of the gut, the heart and the brain, what do these feelings and emotions have to do with reflection? What is it that triggers us to react instinctively to things that we experience with anger, fear, or joy? Why is it sometimes so hard to think logically about things, to critically reflect, when we are so overcome by this tension in the gut, whether it be anger, love, nervousness – or fear?

Emotions can be blinding and misleading. A gut feeling can also be intuitively 'spot on'. A gut feeling can tell you that something is not right, even though it can be hard to put your finger on what it is. For people who have gone through physical, psychological and emotional trauma during childhood the gut feeling can become confused or even silenced. When it involves another person things get much more complicated. How do we know what is what? How do we learn to think before we act? How can we incorporate what we think with what we feel?

> Reflection:
> Can you think of situations where your interpretations
> of experiences have been influenced by
> uncomfortable feelings in the stomach or by love?

We have our feelings, our emotions and our intuition. It is wise to stop, take a breather, and try to take a closer look at why we are reacting the way we do; wait for the water to become clear as stated in the Chines proverb. Often, we need the help and perspective of someone else who might be able to see things differently or from a different angle. This takes us back to the process of reflection that we talked about earlier. Below we suggest a structure for this, to support the process of reflection both individually and together with others.

Reflective format

When we are faced with that which is different and outside of our comfort zone, it is much easier to see our differences and, in particular, the difficulties that different perspectives can entail for our manner of participation and interaction. However, we are often more similar than different and we need to explore why we interpret others the way we do. Thus, in order to understand others and what is affecting their actions and behaviour we need to first understand ourselves, and ourselves in relation to others. This requires reflection or, more specifically, critical reflection.

When Jenny was working as a teacher in a university she developed a reflective format that the students used when on international placements. They found this very valuable. Through the process, they developed a greater appreciation for reflection and a greater understanding of their role in interactions with others (24). The essence of this structure is to encourage a critical reflection about one's own actions, thoughts and feelings. The basis for the reflective process is the story that we tell of what we have experienced, and then we consider this reflectively and critically.

This is done both individually and through reflective dialogue with a peer. The format thus builds on two processes: narrative reflection, "a personal descriptive reflection over experiences", and communicative reflection, "the dialogical reflection over experiences based on a mutual interest of gaining a better understanding of what has been experienced" (25).

The basic structure of this exercise is given over the next two pages, slightly adapted to a more general format that can be used for any situation that one finds troubling or disturbing (26) used with permission of Taylor & Francis, www.tandfonline.com.

Step 1 – Individual narrative reflection

The story: A troubling incident is described in writing. The incident can be anything related to life or work, but it should be something that is challenging or difficult, where you felt misunderstood, or where you did not agree with what was done. The description should be as objective and as detailed as possible.

Narrative reflection: Reflect over this story based on the specific questions below. Write an individual narrative account based on these questions, describing your feelings and experience of the incident.

1. What was the most difficult aspect of this incident? Why?
2. Are there ethical and moral conflicts in the situation, and if so, by whose definition?
3. What was your immediate reaction during the situation? Describe your feelings.
4. Why did you act/respond as you did?
5. How did you interpret the actions of the others in the situation?
6. How did you interpret the manner of communication of the others in the situation?
7. Whose voice and/or perspective is not being heard in the telling of this story?
8. Could this story have been told in a different way?
9. What did you find confusing about the situation or the way the others acted?
10. What would you do if a similar situation arises?
11. What did you learn about yourself?

Step 2 – Communicative reflection with peer

Describe the situation, and your feelings and reactions, to a peer. The peer listens, and then asks questions to stimulate further reflection, for example as below:

1. Describe the critical incident or disorienting dilemma.
2. Describe your actions and immediate feelings.
3. Why did you react in the way you did?
    a. Can you see links to previous experiences, that have affected the way you reacted?
    b. Can you see links to specific views you have of the world, beliefs, that made you react the way you did?
    c. What do you think the other people thought of your way of reacting?
4. Describe what you found confusing about the situation or the other's actions.
5. Describe the ethical issues and difficulties in this dilemma.
6. Why did you identify these? Do you think that the other people involved have the same view as you?
7. What have you learned about yourself?
8. What can we learn from each other?

Step 3– Final individual reflection

Individual reflections: During and after the discussion, consider if there was anything new that you came to understand through discussing critically with your peer. Write this down in a journal. You can return to this and do similar critical reflections at a future time.

> Reflection:
> Take a situation that you have found challenging recently, find a peer, and go through the reflective process described.

We acknowledge that this is an extensive format and process. Learning new skills, or becoming stronger or faster, takes time and effort. To get into the habit of reflecting over experiences also takes practice, so taking the time to do this when faced with particularly challenging situations can be well worthwhile. The process itself can be then simplified and used in daily situations, with the prompt of a few select questions from each step in the process. You may develop other questions that help you. The key is to take a step back and consider the situation and your role in it, from various perspectives, together with others.

To summarise, we need to be critically reflective of ourselves and our actions and of ourselves in relation to what is going on around us. We need to strive to understand each other and it is easier to see ourselves in different perspectives through respectful and reflective dialogue with others. If we cannot start with trying to understand ourselves then we cannot understand others and their actions towards us. As mentioned in the quote at the beginning of this chapter, we sometimes need to wait for the water to become clear, to let things settle, before we can see through the emotional turmoil.

We live in a colourful world. Reflection is imperative for us to see and appreciate the colours around us. What and how we see is dependent on our personal factors, genetic inheritance, experiential history, and what we believe in, amongst others. Similarly, we need reflection to make sense of what we experience. We do this best together with others because we may be 'seeing' things slightly differently. Finally, let's look at how we tie everything together in terms of collaboration.

8 collaboration

CULTURAL REFLECTIVENESS

> No-one can play a game alone.
> One cannot be human by oneself. There is no selfhood
> where there is no community. We do not relate to others
> as the persons we are; we are who we are in relating to others.
>
> James P. Carse (27)

The chapters in this book have described different aspects involved in intercultural collaboration. There are many factors to consider, and a shared practice (or being part of the same system or culture) does not automatically imply collaboration.

There is no easy answer to how to work well together in this dynamic colourful world. What has been suggested in this book is a participatory, communicative, reflective approach. It necessitates an awareness of the challenges involved in terms of the different forces at play in our interactions, who we are and what systems of practices we are a part of.

The base-line is that awareness and understanding of oneself is essential in order to understand others, and this applies to all involved in the collaboration, irrespective of position or status. Our ability to be self-critically reflective and our attitude and approach to each other will make all the difference.

Respectful curiosity

We talked about layers earlier, in chapter 3. When we live together with other people and when we collaborate with others, we need to allow people to show more than their outer layer. This takes time and respect. Respect your layers, and those of others, but also, be curious. What lies under the surface? Who is this person and what is their story?

When we participate in situations together with other people with a curious and respectful attitude, it can allow a number of things to happen. We can learn more about ourselves and about the world around us. But a balanced collaboration requires that we all have the mutual attitude that creates a safe space and allows us to expose and share our layers. This won't always happen: we can be responsible for our own attitude, our own will to reflect, but we can never force others to do something they do not want – or feel the need – to do.

> Reflection:
> Think of a situation where you feel that
> you were not understood; where you felt judged based
> on others seeming to have a superficial understanding of you,
> or where you might have judged someone else hastily.

We do not need to agree with others views in order to respect them as human beings (with a right to their own opinions and beliefs). This respectful curiosity will shine through in how you ask questions and how you treat others. This is part of cultural reflectiveness.

Cultural reflectiveness

Participation. Communication. Reflection. These are interlinked and interdependent in the process of collaboration.

Ultimately, they are dependent on the attitude with which you engage in life and in others. Together with a respectful and curious attitude, we can develop our cultural reflectiveness.

Based on what has been said earlier, cultural reflectiveness is a spin-off from cultural competency and a dissatisfaction with this term. Although we have both used the term cultural competency previously, and it is a term commonly used in literature about culture and intercultural practice and collaboration, we have specifically chosen not to use it. In our view, we can never be culturally competent. Despite its various definitions, the term is, in essence, a contradiction.

We can become more competent at being sensitive to cultural factors. We can become better at listening to, and learning from, people around us. We can become better at reflecting over our reactions to things we do not understand. We can learn more about different cultures and so forth. But as we have seen, cultures are dynamic and always in interaction with each individual. Therefore, we can never be truly culturally competent.

We will instead use the term cultural reflectiveness, which includes cultural sensitivity, cultural awareness and cultural understanding. Cultural reflectiveness is not an end goal or learning outcome, it is a continuous process that develops through lived and reflective experience together with others. It is the capacity to be continuously and critically reflective over one's own manner of participation and collaboration with people from cultures and practices different from our own.

Taking this further, the context we are in, our perspective and that of the person we are conversing with, will affect how culturally reflective we are able to be in any given situation and to what extent we are perceived as such. Who establishes how culturally reflective we are? We ourselves might perceive that we are more or less culturally reflective. This is based on our understanding of the other's culture and of ourselves in relation to this culture. We may not be as culturally reflective as we think. We base our understanding of how suitable our actions are based on how we perceive they are received. However, when communicating inter-culturally as discussed before, we may be basing our understandings on meanings that we have construed and that were not intended. Thus, cultural reflectiveness must consider the perspectives of both others and oneself, situated within a particular context and practice. To help in this process we have suggested the reflective format in the previous chapter.

Playing games

Finally, to collaborate with others we need others. We live in a diverse world with an amazing mix of people, races, cultures, practices and systems. These have always changed and will keep changing. We will keep changing. This is a natural order in the world. Things change. Resisting change can be the short-term easy goal, but with this approach we will stay where we are. We will not grow. We cannot live in this world alone and we cannot collaborate by ourselves.

As children, Fatumo and Jenny both used to play different clapping games with their friends, where they would face each other and clap their hands together according to specific patterns and rhythms that accompanied various singing rhymes. It took practice to learn the routines that went with each rhyme. Some of the kids were easier to coordinate with than others, but it was particularly the ability to adapt to each other's skills that made for a well-coordinated clapping rhyme. This may be a simple metaphor but it exemplifies the point: we cannot play this game of social living and collaboration by ourselves. We need to do it together with others and we need to listen to the other person. This is easier said than done when we have different rhymes and rhythms to our actions and intentions. But irrespective of where we are from, we all have hands, and with mutual will and effort we can learn each other's rhymes and rhythms and even create new ones.

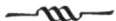

9 conclusion

CROSSING BORDERS

> Meaning is in the living, not simply in
> the thinking or feeling. And it seems to me that
> living well is mostly about loving well ...
> Correct answers can rarely be given.
> We can, though, be conscious of the questions
> so that we can live ourselves into the answers,
> into what in retrospect can be right living.
>
> James Orbinski (28)

We are constantly and unconsciously negotiating borders with those around us. Borders can give structure, help organise our world. However, we cannot let these borders separate us, or be markers of value or of power. Let us not create borders based on fear. We cross borders and we open borders and we all have a responsibility for doing this in respectful and constructive ways.

We believe that (despite all the words written in this book) it all boils down to one simple rule of human interaction: we can never hope to understand anyone else or their practices unless we first start with ourselves. We need to understand who we are and why, and what makes us act the way we do. We need to face our own fears and the fear of seeing sides of ourselves that we are not proud of. We need to explore aspects of ourselves that are difficult and uncomfortable, and take responsibility for our actions. We need to understand our own borders. All this will colour how we interpret others' actions and the judgments we make.

All of us have our own perspectives and practices that have been shaped and formed by our cultural systems of practices, circumstances and the different people who have crossed our paths. Every individual sees the world in different colours depending on their perspective. We can never see the colours that others see but we can appreciate and respect the diversity of the palette. Participating in the lives of other people, with the inevitable ups and downs, is an intricate business and a moral endeavour. Moving outside of our comfort zone, becoming involved in others' concerns will include challenges and can lead to personal discomforts and sacrifices. Yet this is also a privilege.

Care should be taken to acknowledge the myriad of understandings that are – sometimes unconsciously – being communicated under the surface, under the layer we expose to the world and which cannot be immediately understood when viewed from an outsider's perspective. There must be a sincere sensitivity to the differences in communication and culture with attitudes of mutual respect and trust forming the basis for collaboration.

Do not be afraid of differences. Through reflective communication over different opinions we have the potential to learn from each other, to grow as individuals and as professionals. We have the potential to deepen our understanding of each other and of the complexity and diversity of this world. Coming from different backgrounds and contexts can be the catalyst that pushes us to look beyond what we thought we knew. There is potential for considerable development as we live and learn together, coming from different perspectives and ways of viewing the world. Through critically reflective dialogue and action with others, no matter where we are from, we can collaboratively question what we thought we knew and come out as stronger, more empathic individuals and professionals.

epilogue

A COLOURFUL WORLD

> Encouraging self-critical reflection, but not dominating it, matters. So does the explicit recognition that we are here to do good in a practical way in the world as part of our moral self-fashioning. To accomplish that, we need to risk openness to being changed by others.
>
> Arthur Kleinman (29)

By now, we hope you have some new thoughts and ideas about your own life and world, your own practices and state of being, your interactions with those around you. We hope you feel inspired to use all the colours in the rainbow.

Jenny started writing this book a few years ago but then put it on the shelf as she felt she was not ready. We, Fatumo and Jenny, then joined forces, and together we have come this far. Neither of us is probably ready now, and we never will be; every experience brings new insight, new perspectives. Even since we started writing this book, things have changed. We have changed. We have made mistakes. We have learned. A common saying states that "the more you learn, the more you realise what you don't know".

The further down the road we have come, the more we realise the complexity of the contexts we have been in and the naivety of many choices we've made. The more we learn, personally and professionally, the more we are able to reflect upon our experiences and gain new insights into those experiences. The more we learn about ourselves, the more we are able to see why things turned out the way they did based on our expectations, beliefs and attitudes, experience and competence. The cycle of reflection could go on forever!

Having said this, the real issue in collaboration is not how much you reflect, but what this reflection means in practice, how respectful you are with others in thought and action. If we are to live together and function together in a system, we need a language of shared concepts. We need to be more curious about the world around us. The developments in medicine and technology and science would never have come about if there were not people out there who were curious about the world and its functions, about the people in it; people who took crazy chances and rolled with the punches.

We need respect for ourselves and for each other. We need reflective communication and a will to try to learn from each other. We need to realize that the world is changing and we need to be open to the possibility of changing with it.

Thus, to sum it all up. Be respectfully curious. Be critically and constructively reflective.

Be colourful.

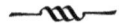

gratitude

TACK, SHUKRAN, MAHADSANID, TASHAKOR, GRMA, MEHRBANI, THANK YOU

There are so many people who have been a part of our lives and who have given us experiences – both good and difficult – that ultimately have let us gain a better understanding of ourselves, and of this world we live in. To all of you, we are immensely grateful. Also, as the saying goes, we stand on the shoulders of giants. Although we do not know you, we are very grateful to all the authors and researchers who have inspired us and taught us, with your words. Our ideas would have been much thinner without you.

We'd like to thank a number of people who have given valuable feedback on the content and structure of this book – in no particular order: Kerstin Erlandsson, Jonas Stier, DT, Aliyu Ndanusa, Charissa Deen, Joel Gonsky and Sagal Shire. We want to thank Helena Mulkerns, for patient support with all our questions, and for wanting to publish this book! Thank you Alisdair Miller for the wonderful photograph on the cover.

We both also have some people that we personally want to mention and thank:

Jenny:

Mam, Pap, Ester, Marcus and Anna: Thank you for never questioning my crazy ideas and my notions of traveling to rather unexpected places. For supporting me and encouraging me and believing in me fully and completely. Tack, for always being there – mer än jag kan säga och av hela mitt hjärta.

To my various teachers and boarding parents in school, I was fortunate indeed to have so many who looked out for me while growing up. To all you wonderful friends I have made in various corners of the world, you have made each place I've lived in home and you are living proof that we all can live and learn together irrespective of where we come from. I wish I could mention you all by name, and I wish I could have you all in the same place! Debbie Rupe, you are a wonder of support and care, thank you for always being there, even though we don't get to meet nearly as often as would be preferable! Susanne Rosberg, your support and belief in me got me through my doctoral studies – without all I learned in that process I would not be the person I am today.

Fatumo:

My role model and Mam, my down-to-earth husband Liibaan, and my children Abdulahi, Juweria and Ahmed: thank you for always believing in me and letting me cross borders both within myself and outside the world. Encouraging me to contribute to the world and to make it a better and colourful place. Ilaahay igama kiin qaado! Love you from the bottom of my heart. To my uncle Hussein who taught me to critically reflect and never be satisfied with only one explanation or perspective and look into different perspectives, uncle, you have always been my role model. To my best friend Sagal, the only person who knows me in-depth, thank you for always being there for me, may we grow old together and enjoy our rocking chairs side by side. Kerstin Erlandsson and Sonia Bentling, thank you *for introducing me to the field of intercultural and transcultural. You are the teachers, colleagues and friends I look up to and I have learned so much from you.*

Finally, we want to thank you, the reader, for taking part of the stories and ponderings of this book. We hope you have come to the end with further thoughts about what it means to live and learn together. May your journey be colourful and full of reflections!

Chapter notes

Please find the reference notes for each chapter below:

chapter 1: introduction

(1) Crichton, M. (2005). *State of fear*. London: Harper-Collins, p.678.

(2) Wickford, J. (2010). *Physiotherapists in Afghanistan. Exploring, encouraging and experiencing professional development in the Afghan development context*. (Doctoral dissertation), University of Gothenburg, Gothenburg.

(3) Gibran, K. (2011). *The treasured writings of Kahlil Gibran*. New York: Philosophical Library, p.20.

(4) Tolkien, J.R.R. (1954). *The fellowship of the ring*. London: George Allen & Unwin, p.60.

(5) Hofstede, G. (2001). *Culture's consequences: comparing values, behaviors, institutions, and organizations across nations* (2. ed.). Thousand Oaks: Sage, p.10.

(6) https://en.oxforddictionaries.com/definition/practice

(7) https://en.oxforddictionaries.com/definition/system

chapter 2: context

(8) Hall, S. (1976). *Beyond culture*. New York: Doubleday.

chapter 3: person

(9) Mezirow, J. (1991). *Transformative dimensions of adult learning* (1st ed.). San Francisco: Jossey-Bass.

(10) Wickford, J., & Svensson, Ali E. (2016). *Colour in grey - expressions of (be)longing*. A collection of poetry and artwork.

chapter 4: pushing, pulling or status quo?

(11) Herbert, F. (1965). *Dune*. London: NEL Books, p.220.

(12) https://en.oxforddictionaries.com/definition/power

(13) Hofstede, G. (2001). *Culture's consequences: comparing values, behaviors, institutions, and organizations across nations* (2nd ed.). Thousand Oaks: Sage.

(14) Osman, F., Klingberg-Allvin, M., Flacking, R. and Schön, U.K., 2016. Parenthood in transition – Somali-born parents' experiences of and needs for parenting support programs. *BMC International Health and Human Rights*. 16(7). 1-11.

chapter 5: participation

(15) Wenger, E. (1998). *Communities of practice: learning, meaning and identity*. Cambridge: Cambridge University Press, p.4.

(16) Lave, J. & Wenger, E. (1991). *Situated learning. Legitimate peripheral participation*. Cambridge: Cambridge University Press.

(17) Hayward, C., Simpson, L., & Wood, L. (2004). Still Left out in the Cold: Problematising Participatory Research and Development. *Sociologia Ruralis, 44(1)*, 95-108, p.98.

(18) Wickford, J., & Rosberg, S. (2012). From idealistic helper to enterprising learner: critical reflections on personal development through experiences from Afghanistan. *Physiotherapy Theory and Practice, 28(4)*, 283-291.

(19) Wickford, J. (2014). Conscious seeing: A description of a reflective framework used with final-year Swedish physiotherapy students in the context of international clinical placements. *European Journal of Physiotherapy, 16*, 41-48, p.42.

chapter 6: communication

(20) Hall, S. (1976). *Beyond culture*. New York: Doubleday.

(21) Wickford, J. (2014). Conscious seeing: A description of a reflective framework used with final-year Swedish physiotherapy students in the context of international clinical placements. *European Journal of Physiotherapy, 16*, 41-48. p.42.

chapter 7: reflection

(22) Rogers, R. (2001). Reflection in higher education: A concept analysis. *Innovative Higher Education*, 26(1), 37-57, p.41.

(23) Mezirow, J. (1990). How critical reflection triggers transformative learning. In J. Mezirow (Ed.), *Fostering critical reflection in adulthood: a guide to transformative and emancipatory learning* (pp. 1-20). San Francisco: Jossey-Bass Publishers, p.1.

(24) Wickford, J. (2014). Conscious seeing: A description of a reflective framework used with final-year Swedish physiotherapy students in the context of international clinical placements. *European Journal of Physiotherapy, 16*, p.41-48.

(25) Wickford, J. (2014). Conscious seeing: A description of a reflective framework used with final-year Swedish physiotherapy students in the context of international clinical placements. *European Journal of Physiotherapy, 16*, p.42.

(26) Basic reflective framework. Adapted from: Wickford, J. (2014). Conscious seeing: A description of a reflective framework used with final-year Swedish physiotherapy students in the context of international clinical placements. *European Journal of Physiotherapy, 16*, 41-48, p.43. Used with permission from Taylor & Francis, www.tandfonline.com

chapter 8: collaboration

(27) Carse, J. P. (1986). *Finite and infinite games. A vision of life as play and possibility*. New York: Ballantine Books, p.45.

chapter 9: closing thoughts

(28) Orbinski, J. (2009). *An imperfect offering: Humanitarian action in the twenty-first century.* London: Rider, p.32.

(29) Kleinman, A. (2006). *What really matters: living a moral life amidst uncertainty and danger.* Oxford: Oxford University Press, p.194.

Bibliography and recommended reading

Below is a list of some of the references that have inspired us through the years, and on which we have built various ideas presented in the book. We acknowledge the great contribution these authors have made, and are grateful for all we have learned from them!

Biggs, J., & Tang, C. (2011). *Teaching for quality learning at university* (4th ed.). Maidenhead: McGraw-Hill/Society for Research into Higher Education.

Billett, S. (2004). Workplace participatory practices – conceptualising workplace as learning environments. *Journal of Workplace Learning, 16*(6), 312-324.

Brookfield, S. (1990). Using critical incidents to explore learners' assumptions. In J. Mezirow (Ed.), *Fostering critical reflection in adulthood. A guide to transformative and emancipatory learning* (pp. 177-193). San Fransisco: Jossey-Bass.

Buber, M. (1990). *Jag och du* (2nd ed.). Falun: Dualis Förlag AB.

Campinha-Bacote, J. (2003). *The process of cultural competence in the delivery of healthcare services: A culturally competent model of care*: Transcultural CARE Associates.

Carse, J. P. (1986). *Finite and infinite games. A vision of life as play and possibility.* New York: Ballantine Books.

Doidge, N. (2007). *The brain that changes itself.* London: Penguin Books.

Dunn, B. D., Galton, H. C., Morgan, R., Evans, D., Oliver, C., Dalgleish, T. (2010). "Listening to your heart: how interoception shapes emotion experience and intuitive decision making". *Psychological Science,* 21(12), 1835-1844.

Eriksson-Baaz, M. (2005). *The paternalism of partnership: a postcolonial reading of identity in development aid.* London: Zed Books

Freire, P. (1998). *Pedagogy of freedom : ethics, democracy, and civic courage.* Lanham, Md. ; Oxford: Rowman & Littlefield.

Freire, P. (2005). *Pedagogy of the oppressed* (30th anniversary ed.). New York: Continuum International Publishing Group.

Gershon, M. D. (1999). *The second brain.* New York: Harper.

Hall, E. (1966). *The hidden dimension.* New York: Doubleday.

Hall, S. (1976). *Beyond culture.* New York: Doubleday.

Harrod Buhner, S. (2004). *The secret teachings of plants. The intelligence of the heart in the direct perception of nature.* Vermont: Bear & Company.

Hofstede, G. (2001). *Culture's consequences: comparing values, behaviors, institutions, and organizations across nations* (2nd ed.). Thousand Oaks: Sage.

Illeris, K. (2009). A comprehensive understanding of human learning. In K. Illeris (Ed.), *Contemporary theories of learning. Learning theorists ... in their own words* (pp. 7-19). Oxon: Routledge.

Kleinman, A. (2006). *What really matters: living a moral life amidst uncertainty and danger*. Oxford: Oxford University Press.

Lave, J. (2009). "The practice of learning". In K. Illeris (Ed.), *Contemporary theories of learning: Learning theorists ... in their own words* (pp. 200-208). Oxon: Routledge.

Lave, J., & Wenger, E. (1991). *Situated learning. Legitimate peripheral participation*. Cambridge: Cambridge University Press.

McDonald-Gibson, C. (2016). *Cast away. Stories of survival from Europe's refugee crisis*. London: Portobello Books.

Mezirow, J. (1990). *Fostering critical reflection in adulthood: a guide to transformative and emancipatory learning* (1st ed.). San Francisco: Jossey-Bass Publishers.

Mezirow, J. (1991). *Transformative dimensions of adult learning* (1st ed.). San Francisco: Jossey-Bass.

Orrenius, N. (2012). *Sverige forever in my heart*. Stockholm: Natur & Kultur.

Osman, F., Klingberg-Allvin, M., Flacking, R., & Schön, U.-K. (2016). "Parenthood in transition–Somali-born parents' experiences of and needs for parenting support programmes". *BMC international health and human rights*, 16(1), 1-11.

Sacks, O. (2011). *The mind's eye*. London: Picador.

Stier, J. (2004). *Kulturmöten - en introduktion till interkulturella studier*. Lund: Studentlitteratur.

Susskind, L., & Hrabovsky, G. (2013). *Classical mechanics - the theoretical minimum*. London: Penguin Books.

Svensson, G. (2011). *Mordförsök på tilliten. En bok om tortyr*. Stockholm: Carlsson Bokförlag & Svenska Röda Korset.

Wenger, E. (1998). *Communities of practice: learning, meaning and identity*. Cambridge: Cambridge University Press.

Wickford, J. (2010). *Physiotherapists in Afghanistan. Exploring, encouraging and experiencing professional development in the Afghan development context*. (Doctoral dissertation), University of Gothenburg, Gothenburg.

Wickford, J. (2014). "Conscious seeing: A description of a reflective framework used with final-year Swedish physiotherapy students in the context of international clinical placements". *European Journal of Physiotherapy, 16*, 41-48.

Wickford, J., & Rosberg, S. (2012). "From idealistic helper to enterprising learner: critical reflections on personal development through experiences from Afghanistan". *Physiotherapy Theory and Practice, 28*(4), 283-291.

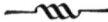

– fin –

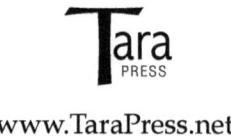

www.TaraPress.net

www.ingramcontent.com/pod-product-compliance
Lightning Source LLC
Chambersburg PA
CBHW031156020426
42333CB00013B/690